Intermittent Fasting for Women

Proven Techniques to Lose Weight, Autophagy, Reset Your Body and Deny Aging

Melissa May

Your Free Gift

Before you go any further, why not pick up a free gift from me to you?

WEIGHT LOSS QUIZ

If you're a woman interested in trying intermittent fasting to achieve your weight loss goals, it's essential to find the right number of calories for you to eat in order to see success. The good news is that you can easily determine the exact number of calories you need to eat based on your metabolism, activity level, and time frame using our quiz at the link provided. Simply follow the prompts and you'll have all the details you need to get started on your weight loss journey with intermittent fasting.

Scan here to learn how much you need to eat in order to achieve your goals.

Table of Contents

Introduction

Did you know that intermittent fasting can assist you in losing weight? Do you want to get stronger while simultaneously shedding those excess pounds? If that's the case, you've come to the correctplace. Both of those benefits can be achieved through the practice of intermittent fasting. But that's not the only thing it's capable of. The benefits of intermittent fasting extend far beyond the realm of simple weight loss, including the improvement of the immune system and the prevention of inflammation. You read it correctly, ladies: missing meals can be beneficial to your overall health.

In this book, I will attempt to explain the science behind intermittent fasting and how it can be used to achieve your desired goals being a woman. I will cover topics such as the types of intermittent fasting, the benefits and risks of using it, and how to get started with the practice. Allof the information is presented in an easy-to-understand way so that everyone can benefit from it. So if you're looking for an effective way to lose weight and improve your health, look no furtherthan intermittent fasting.

It can be noted that as the popularity of intermittent fasting continues to skyrocket, an increasing number of individuals who appear to have tried a variety of diets without any discernible results are pondering the question of whether or not the novel approach to weight loss might be effective for them. Not only is it common because of the various advantages that one is able to take advantage of during the process of intermittent fasting, but also the fact that fasting is more adaptable and natural makes it something that many people prefer. Intermittent fasting has become very popular in recent years. People who have attempted traditional ways of dieting sometimes find restricting their meal options and measuring the number of calories they consume to be extremely overwhelming.

The fact that one can experience weight reduction in addition to other benefits of intermittent fasting without having to worry about regaining the lost weight again is what makes this method really impressive and something that is definitely worth trying out. The fasting methods are very simple to put into practice, and the fact that you don't have to worry too much about the meals you're allowed to consume during the eating window is one of the reasons why the procedure is so tempting. Fasting can be beneficial for a variety of health reasons. The ability of the body to transition into fat-burning mode as a result of intermittent fasting is one of the things that contribute to its efficacy as a method for weight loss. This, in turn, leads to a reduction in abdominal fat.

When the body is in the process of burning fat, the cells in the body become more sensitive to insulin, and at the same time, the production of human growth hormone also rises. This book has described in depth some of the benefits that one gets to experience as a result of practicing intermittent fasting, and practicing intermittent fasting comes with a number of benefits. You will find all the information that you need to know in order to not only get started but also get to realize success with intermittent fasting, regardless of whether you are already well-versed in intermittent fasting and all that it entails or are just getting started. This applies whether you are just getting started or whether you are already well-versed in intermittent fasting and all that it entails.

Skipping meals on purpose can help enhance mental clarity, lower the risk of type 2 diabetes, heart disease, and fat gain, and protect you from acquiring neurodegenerative disorders like Alzheimer's disease and dementia. Skipping meals also helps balance your blood sugar and insulin levels. In addition, if you are interested in delaying the effects of aging on your body, intermittent fasting may be of assistance. Your cells will experience a brief period of stress as a result of intermittent fasting; however, as your body becomes accustomed to managing stress over time, it will become better able to delay the aging process by more effectively repairing physical injuries, warding off disease, and gaining muscle mass.

One of the most compelling pieces of evidence supporting the effectiveness of intermittent fastingwas the CALERIE study. The

Comprehensive Assessment of the Long-term Effects of Reducing Intake of Energy (CALERIE) study was conducted over a two-year period and involved over 200 people who followed either intermittent fasting or a continuous calorie restriction diet.

The results of the CALERIE study showed that people following an intermittent fasting diet lost more body fat and had improved metabolic health, compared to those following a continuous calorie restriction diet. Furthermore, the participants on the intermittent fasting diet reported greater adherence to their diet, suggesting that the diet is easier to maintain over time.

These findings have been supported by numerous other studies, which have demonstrated that intermittent fasting is an effective way to reduce body fat, improve metabolic health, and even extend lifespan.

As is the case with any topic pertaining to nutrition and food, it is vital that you educate yourself on the fundamentals, as well as the requirements of your unique body, and that you conduct research and trials to determine which eating strategy is best for you. No matter what your motivations are for fasting, this book will provide you with all of the information you want to achieve your goals successfully. You are going to acquire more information regarding each of the followingcommon types of fasting:

• 16/8 Time-restricted intermittent fasting – Do not consume any food or liquids for sixteen hours, and only eat during the remaining eight hours of the day.

• Eat-stop-eat intermittent fasting - Eat normally for the first five days of each week and thenrefrain from eating for the remaining two days of the week.

• 5:2 intermittent fasting - Maintain a normal eating schedule for five days of the week, andon the remaining two days, have two meals per day.

• Alternate day intermittent fasting: Instead of eating three meals per day, try eating twomeals on some days and three meals on others.

• The warrior intermittent fasting plan: The warrior plan involves eating only one meal perday and fasting for the remaining 23 hours.

So girls, if you are looking for an effective diet strategy to help you reduce body fat, improve metabolic health, and extend your lifespan, then you need to read this book. It will provide you with an in-depth look at intermittent fasting to help you understand how it works and how to successfully incorporate it into your lifestyle. So don't wait any longer and start reading!

Chapter 1

Fitness and Intermittent Fasting

Many people are interested in gaining a better understanding of what exactly is involved in the practice of intermittent fasting as it is progressively becoming more popular and has become a hot topic in the realm of nutrition. People now have access to an efficient form of dieting known as intermittent fasting, which may still be used by them even if their schedules are extremely packed and hectic. It is essential, in order to achieve success with an intermittent diet, to have an understanding of what the diet comprises. Due to the fact that there are a great number of dietaryvariants, it may be of great use to find a good resource that not only helps one to create lean muscle but also gets to burn fat while doing so. This is because there are a great number of dietary variations.

When you practice intermittent fasting, you don't have to stop what you're doing every two to threehours to have a meal as you would if you were doing traditional fasting. You are not obligated toforce yourself to eat at specific times throughout the day; rather, you are free to choose when andhow you want to eat. Although it is sometimes referred to as a diet, intermittent fasting is actuallymore accurately described as a dieting approach that can also be considered a lifestyle. Becausethere is so little information provided about the meals that one should eat and the requisite ratio, intermittent fasting cannot be properly recognized to be a diet. Diets are intended to provide specific information about the foods that one should eat. It does, however, indicate an extreme way of thinking about the appropriate times for eating.

What exactly does it mean to fast intermittently?

The practice of going without food or drink for a predetermined amount of time is the cornerstone of the intermittent fasting method, which has been around for quite some time. It is also a patternof eating in which one alternates between times of eating and periods of fasting over the course of a certain amount of time. It is important to note that intermittent fasting is not a diet in and of itself but rather a pattern of eating in which an individual deliberately skips some meals. It meansthat one consumes calories at a specific period within the day, and then refrains from taking in any food for the majority of the remaining 24 hours of the day. The practice of intermittent fastingcomes with a variety of health benefits, and regardless of whether or not you intend to fully adoptthe dieting pattern, you can still benefit in some way from this emerging health trend.

The practice of intermittent fasting is becoming increasingly popular, particularly among celebrities, who are embracing the health trend for the purpose of achieving weight loss,improving their health, and enhancing their cognitive abilities. When you cut down on the amountof time you spend eating each meal, you may make the time you do spend eating have more of a purpose. The main focus of intermittent fasting is not on the kinds of foods that one should consume or those that one should steer clear of; rather, it is on the times of day when such foodscan be consumed. The vast majority of people get to experience fasting every day while they are asleep, and practicing intermittent fasting can be as easy as extending the period of time during which one is fasting. You have the option of skipping breakfast and then eating the first meal and the second sometime between 4 and 8 o'clock in the evening.

It is recommended that one first acquire some fundamental knowledge regarding the practice of fasting in order to have a clear understanding of what is involved in intermittent fasting. You might also choose to limit the amount of time you eat throughout your fast to eight hours, which would result in a daily fast of 16 hours. Additionally, this is the most common form of intermittent fasting technique.

Many individuals may be under the impression that observing an intermittent fast is complicated or difficult to undertake, however, this is not the case. During the fasting time, many people report having greater energy and generally feeling better than before.

During the period of fasting, one is not permitted to consume any food; nevertheless, they are permitted to drink beverages such as water, coffee, or any other beverages that do not contain calories. During the fasting phase, itis possible to consume limited quantities of meals low in calories according to certain variations of the intermittent fasting method. Intake of supplements is also permitted so long as these supplements do not contain any calories.

1.1 A Concise History of the Practice of Intermittent Fasting

Fasting on an intermittent basis is not a novel concept; in fact, many communities of people all over the world have been engaging in this type of eating restriction since the beginning of recorded history. Since the beginning of human history, people have found it necessary, at times, to deprivethemselves of food because there was none available for consumption. This practice has continued for thousands of years. There are documented cases in which individuals have chosento abstain from food entirely for religious reasons. Many world faiths, including Christianity, Buddhism, and Islam, require their followers to observe fasting during certain times of the year. People have a natural tendency to restrict their food intake when they are ill.

When you browse through the books on religion and ethnology, you'll find fascinating descriptions of the many various kinds of fasting practices and forms that people engaged in during different eras. There has recently been a resurgence in people's interest in the practice of fasting, which may be attributed to a number of well-known books and dietary advice that have discussed the several advantages that can be attained through the practice. There are a number of books that tend to encourage different types of fasting diets, each with its own set of potential health benefits. There are also a great number of websites and blogs available online that provide information pertaining to fasting; nevertheless, the health benefits that have been scientifically verified are based on some observational data that was carried out on religious fasting.

The majority of the material that is now accessible on intermittent fasting, including the evidencethat demonstrates the positive effects that fasting has on one's health, is based on research thatwas carried out on animal models. Changes in weight and metabolism, cardiovascular disease, type 2 diabetes, and cancer are among the documented health consequences that have been related to these changes. In addition, there are research findings that have examined the practice of intermittent fasting in humans, and evidence has been produced that analyzes the influence that intermittent fasting has on the health of individuals. There is nothing inherently abnormal or

unnatural about fasting, and the human body is designed to be able to tolerate the extended periods of time during which one may go without eating while fasting.

When compared to dieting, fasting may appear to be relatively straightforward and uncomplicateddue to the fact that it has always been practiced. The practice of skipping meals, such as breakfastor even lunch, is one of the most common forms of unintentional intermittent fasting. Our predecessors historically engaged in activities such as hunting and gathering, and because of this, they were always in a state of fasting while they searched for sustenance. When there was a lack of food or when the seasons changed, fasting continued to be a prominent part of the waypeople lived their lives, despite the advent of agriculture and the subsequent rise of civilization.

Before irrigation became widespread, a lack of rain frequently meant famine. As a result, peoplefrequently engaged in periods of fasting to ensure that their preserved food would last for longer periods of time. People also stored grain and meat that had been cured for consumption during the winter. In addition, fasting is mandated by many religions; nevertheless, each faith, including Judaism, Christianity, Islam, and Hinduism, amongst others, has its own distinctive approach to the practice of fasting.

The practice of fasting is not only highly helpful and stimulating, but it is also the best thing for one's overall health. Fasting for an extended period of time has a tendency to cause changes in all of the body's processes. Fasting causes considerable reductions in both the blood sugar and insulin levels of the person doing the fasting, in addition to an increase in the production of hormones. Because one is able to both reduce the number of calories consumed and increase the rate at which fat is burned, intermittent fasting is one of the simplest methods that lead to weight loss. Because of this, having a solid understanding of the many types of fasting can help bring about clarity and provide additional insight into the topic of intermittent fasting;

1.2 Different kinds of fasting

If you are familiar with the various forms of fasting, you will have a better understanding of what intermittent fasting entails and will be able to communicate this concept more clearly. The following is a list of some of the various forms of fasting:

Alternate day fasting is a sort of fasting that requires the practitioner to observe fasting days, during which they abstain from consuming any meals or beverages that contain energy. It is a less structured eating pattern in which one alternates between periods of not consuming any calories and periods in which they do consume food. On the days that they are not abstaining from food, some people continue the practice by adhering to a ketogenic or high-fat diet. On the other hand, there are individuals who adhere to a well-balanced meal plan on the days that theyare to consume food. This sort of fasting, when properly observed, has been shown to be just assuccessful as lowering one's calorie intake, and it also brings about a reduction in the amount ofplasma cholesterol and triglycerides.

It was discovered that fasting every other day was beneficial for weight loss as well as an improvement in metabolism. Additionally, it has been demonstrated that this particular form of fasting enhances the performance of important organs.

Time-restricted feeding is a technique of fasting that involves abstaining from food consumptionbetween 12 and 16 hours per day, after which you are allowed to consume food for the remaining8 hours of the day. Because it does not result in negative conditions such as exhaustion, anger, disorientation, and sadness, amongst other negative difficulties, this sort of fasting is advocated in large part because it does not result in these conditions. The majority of people who practice this form of fasting do so by omitting breakfast in the morning and waiting until approximately lunchtime to consume their first meal of the day. They are then able to remain there for approximately seven hours until they need to eat again the following day.

The practice of abstaining from food and drink in accordance with one's religious beliefs is knownas fasting, and it is done with the purpose of gaining both bodily and spiritual advantages. The Islamic kind of fasting does not involve the restriction of energy; yet, because fasting can vary between 11 and 22 hours, the decreased intake of fluids and foods ends up modifying the body in a variety of ways, and it is possible that weight reduction will be attained.

People who regularly observe different types of religious fasting typically experience significant weight loss, along with lower levels of glucose in their blood when fasting and a lower incidence of diabetes.

Modified fasting is a form of fasting in which the individual consumes around 25% of the recommended daily calorie needs for a period of two days, after which they are permitted to eat normally for a period of five days.

1.3 Busting Fasting Myths

In spite of the fact that intermittent fasting is currently receiving a lot of attention in the media, there are still a lot of individuals who are unsure as to whether or not the diet pattern is beneficial,secure, and healthful. There are many myths that have developed around the practice of intermittent fasting, and if one does not have a good understanding of the pattern of eating that itentails, one may not be able to reap the benefits that come along with it.

Some of the common misunderstandings are as follows:

Weight loss has been linked to intermittent fasting; however, this is only the case for individuals who both devote time to fasting and consume fewer calories overall.

It is vital to keep in mind that one can still lose weight even if they eat as much as they like as long as they practice intermittent fasting. Although the majority of people who practice intermittent fasting end up eating less food than they did before, this is not always the case. Even if someonedoes not lower the total number of calories that they consume in a given day, engaging in intermittent fasting can still result in weight loss and the loss of fat. This is due to the fact that intermittent fasting helps reduce inflammation in the body, which is one of the primary factors that contribute to weight gain. When a person engages in fasting, there is an improvement in glucosemetabolism, and there is also an increase in sensitivity to insulin.

During your fasting periods, you are not allowed to consume anything.

There is a widespread misconception that while one is fasting, one must abstain from eating or drinking anything. If you are participating in intermittent fasting, then you must continue to drink water throughout the fasting period; however, water may not be the only thing that you are allowedto ingest during this time. One of the most significant advantages of practicing intermittent fastingis that it allows you to lengthen the period of time during which your body is in a state characterizedby low levels of insulin.

It is possible that you will be permitted to consume beverages like coffee that do not trigger insulin production, as well as a small amount of fat that is able to maintain the body in a ketotic condition. After that, it may be of assistance in the process of shedding fat and producing fuel for the metabolism.

The best method of fasting is alternate-day fasting.

There are many different variations of the intermittent fasting method. There is a form of fasting known as alternate-day fasting, in which participants are required to severely limit their caloric intake to less than 500 calories, all of which must be ingested at one meal, and the practice mustbe maintained continuously. The 5:2 fast requires following a normal eating schedule for the firstfive days of the diet, after which participants are instructed to drastically reduce their calorie consumption for the final two days. The 16/8 method of fasting requires abstaining from food for 16 hours, after which a window of 8 hours is allotted for eating.

Although 16:8 fasting is one of the easiest dieting patterns that can be practiced daily, particularlywith a doctor's approval, alternate-day fasting is one of the easiest dieting patterns that can be practiced occasionally to enhance weight loss and also contribute to cardiovascular health. Alternate-day fasting can be adopted occasionally to enhance weight loss and also contribute to cardiovascular health.

Those who engage in strenuous physical activity are unable to participate in the intermittent fasting diet.

It is imperative that you speak with a medical professional before making any changes to your dietary routine; nonetheless, the fact that you put in a lot of effort at the gym does not give you apass if you want to avoid partaking in intermittent fasting. Even if someone is participating in strenuous physical activity, they may still reap the benefits of intermittent fasting. The person should just plan the exercise and the fasting at suitable times.

It is a starvation diet.

It is not necessarily the case that skipping a meal for a number of hours would result in starvation.Numerous research investigations have shown that a person's metabolic rate will not slow downeven after they have gone without food for sixty consecutive hours. Fasting has been one of the strategies that have enabled many people to make it through times of severe deprivation throughout human history. The condition known as starvation is characterized by extreme pain as a result of hunger. A person who is starving to death typically has their fat stores depleted, which compels the body to break down its own muscular tissue in order to obtain energy.

Through the process of intermittent fasting, the body is able to release energy that had been stored as fat while sparing the lean body tissues and muscles. Intermittent fasting does not havethe capability of affecting lean body tissues, particularly if it is carried out under the advice of a dietician, and this is true even if the individual regularly participates in activities such as running marathons or has a body fat level that is lower than 4%.

You will be famished throughout the entire day.

According to the findings of a number of studies, an individual's feeling of hunger is likely to lessenduring fasting days. Furthermore, after only two weeks of intermittent fasting, obese people havebeen observed to experience decreased hunger, which persisted at a low level. Consuming an adequate number of calories on days when one is not fasting is more of a battle than it is an experience of hunger.

Once you've given intermittent fasting a try, you could find that it becomes a permanentpart of your lifestyle.

When you first begin to practice intermittent fasting, you may notice that your hunger and desireschange. This is one of the many benefits of this method of dieting. You will notice that you no longer want the potato chips or the noon snack once you have abstained from them for a sufficientamount of time, and it will not have been difficult for you to get over the desire to have them.

The primary goal here should be to retrain your taste receptors to only crave good food and to turn away from foods that are more likely to cause weight gain and the development of chronic diseases.

1.4 Maintenance of macronutrients and calorie intake

To be successful with intermittent fasting, one must reduce the number of calories one consumesin order to achieve weight loss and reap some of the benefits that are associated with the diet. Asa result, it is essential to have some understanding of what the macronutrients are in order to accomplish either of these goals. In order for the body to function properly, it is necessary to consume certain macronutrients, which are briefly explained below.

Protein: If you engage in strenuous workouts and exercises despite the fact that you are fasting,then you should have a solid understanding of proteins and the role that they play in the body. Proteins are regarded to be the building blocks for muscles and also help the body recover afterengaging in some strenuous exercise. Protein is very important, and it may be obtained from a wide variety of meals, including meat, beans, dairy products, nuts, and so on. One gram of proteinshould be consumed for every pound that an athlete weighs in order to follow the standard recommendation. Therefore, if you weigh 150 pounds, you want to make it a goal to consume at least 150 grams of protein on a daily basis. Approximately four calories are contained in each gram of food.

Carbohydrates: They are the body's primary source of energy, and they make up the vast majority of the calories that an individual is able to take in on a daily basis. Sugars and starches are both types of carbohydrates, but sugars are generally easier to digest than starches, which allows sugars to be taken into the bloodstream much more quickly. Starches are typically digested over a considerably longer period of time than other types of food, and once the digestion process is complete, the starch is stored as glycogen in the muscles. There are four calories in one gramof carbohydrate, and some of the foods that include carbohydrates, such as grain, bread, pasta, rice, potatoes, and sugar, are examples of sources of calories.

Fats: Fats are also very necessary for the overall health of the body, and generally there are threedifferent types of fats. There is a third type of fat known as Tran's fat, in addition to saturated and unsaturated fats. Because of the refining process, the fats sold by Tran are categorized as "bad" fats, and consuming them may increase the risk of developing a variety of illnesses, including heart disease. Although saturated isn't inherently bad, you should still try to restrict your exposureto them as much as possible. Butter, lard, beef, cream, and other similar items are all examples of foods that contain saturated fat. Because, in addition to their many other positive effects on health, unsaturated fats reduce the likelihood of developing heart disease, making them the typeof fat most often recommended. Foods like avocados, almonds, olive oil, and other things have unsaturated fats that can be consumed by the body.

Caloric Maintenance: The number of calories that the body needs to consume on a daily basis in order to keep itself in a state in which there is neither weight loss nor weight gain is referred toas the "caloric maintenance" number. The number of calories gained is often different for each person, with a greater amount being gained by those who are younger, more physically active, and who also have a greater amount of muscle mass. Carbohydrates, proteins, and lipids, in the right proportions, can provide the necessary calories for the maintenance of body weight. If you want to lose weight, the number of calories you consume each day should be less than the number of calories you burn off in a given day. By making use of calorie calculators that are available online, you are able to ascertain the number of calories that you are able to consume orshed on a daily basis.

Chapter 2

Weight loss with fasting

Fasting enhances virtually every element of your health, both physical and mental. It can help you take charge of your body and your well-being as long as you do it responsibly and attentively. Intermittent fasting can be done in a variety of ways. You must select the strategy that is most effective for you and will help you achieve your health objectives. Sometimes you'll combine methods or experiment until you find one you can stick with.

2.1 A healthy lifestyle

One of the most prevalent motivations for individuals to begin intermittent fasting is weight loss, yet this only touches the surface of the potential benefits. Other than causing you to lose weight, intermittent fasting has a number of health benefits for your body. In addition to this, it assists in the regulation of sugar levels in the blood, the reduction of persistent or widespread inflammation, and the enhancement of the health of the heart.

It has also been found that intermittent fasting improves brain health, which may result in a reduced probability of developing major brain illnesses such as Alzheimer's disease. Last but notleast, there is speculation among certain professionals that it could help in the fight against cancerand increase the efficacy of chemotherapy for patients already afflicted with the disease.

You've definitely heard that if you eat less, you'll lose more weight. However, what if losing weighthas less to do with the quantity of food you're consuming and more to do with the length of time you spend eating it? When you first learn how intermittent fasting works, you might think, "Well, okay, if you eat during a smaller window of time, you'll be eating fewer calories, and that's why you lose weight." However, this is not necessarily the case.

That's a big part of it: in certain instances, you'll be eating fewer calories, particularly due to the fact that you won't be mindlessly nibbling in the middle of the night, which is a habit that can swiftly contribute to weight gain. However, this is only part of the narrative. Studies have demonstrated that the practice of intermittent fasting can lead to weight loss and an improved metabolism evenin the absence of a general reduction in calories consumed.

2.2 Weight loss studies

A study that was published in the journal Translational Research indicated that following a regimen of intermittent fasting can result in a reduction of three to eight percent of total body weight in a period of three to twenty-four weeks. The individuals in this study lost between 4 and7 percent of their waist circumference, which suggests that they shed abdominal fat, also knownas visceral fat, which is the sort of fat that is regarded to be the most detrimental to a person's physical health.

The visceral cavity is the area of the abdominal cavity that stores visceral fat. It is located in closeproximity to a number of important organs, such as the stomach, the pancreas, the intestines,

and the liver. Because it can disrupt your hormones and the way your body works, having a lot ofvisceral fat is more harmful than having additional subcutaneous fat (the fat that lays just underneath your skin). This is because visceral fat can be found deep within the abdominal cavity.There is a correlation between it and an increased likelihood of developing cardiovascular disease, cancer, stroke, diabetes, arthritis, obesity, and depression. There is no foolproof method for determining whether the fat in your body is subcutaneous or visceral, but if you tend to carry most of your weight around your abdominal region, it's likely that you have a higher amount of visceral fat than subcutaneous fat.

People who adhere to dietary programs that provide variety in meal choices, such as intermittent fasting, have been shown in studies to be more successful in sticking to the diet and maintaining weight reduction than those who adhere to strict calorie-control diets. In non-obese women, rigid diets are connected with symptoms of disordered eating as well as a higher body mass index, which is a measurement of your body fat based on your weight and height. Flexible dieting regimens, such as intermittent fasting, are not associated with these symptoms.

It's possible that hearing this would be disheartening, particularly if you've bought into the idea that the only way to lose weight is to reduce the number of calories you eat and increase the amount of exercise you do; nevertheless, this is actually quite encouraging information. You don'tneed to spend your days counting calories, eating too little, and staying away from good fats in order to lose weight. Fasting on an intermittent basis is a more effective strategy. However, it is important to note that while fasting is beneficial for some people, it is not effective for others. It isvital that you locate the method of weight loss that is most effective for you specifically.

2.3 Weight loss myths

The concepts of "eat less and move more" and "calories in versus calories out" are by far the most prevalent and long-lasting approaches to weight loss. If you take a look at the numbers, you'll see that these beliefs don't add up, despite the fact that the general premise that underpinsthese theories is that in order to lose weight, you need to consume fewer calories than you burn off. People have been given advice during the past two decades to adhere to diets that are low in calories and fat and to consume between five and six smaller meals on a daily basis.

Despite this, there has been a significant rise in the prevalence of obesity over the past twenty years. There is an argument that people simply aren't putting in the work required to lose weight,but in many situations, this isn't true. Of course, there is the argument that people simply aren't putting in the work required to lose weight. There are a large number of people who maintain a "healthy" diet and exercise routine, yet they have no visible results to show for it. This is due tothe fact that losing weight is not as easy as it may seem, and popular wisdom has been shownto be incorrect.

During its nearly eight-year duration, the Women's Health Initiative study tracked a total of around fifty thousand female participants. During that time period, one-half of the ladies adhered to a dietthat was reduced in fat and calories and increased the amount of physical activity they did by

14%. This group was referred to as the intervention group throughout the study. The remaining fifty percent of the women continued with their customary schedules of diet and exercise. After almost eight years, the difference in weight loss between the intervention group and the control group was less than 2 pounds on average.

2.4 Tips for success with intermittent fasting

If you're interested in trying intermittent fasting as a weight loss tool, here are a few tips to help you succeed:

- Stay hydrated: It's important to drink plenty of water during your fasting periods to help keep your body hydrated and flush out toxins.

- Eat nutrient-dense foods: During your eating window, focus on filling your plate with nutrient-dense foods such as vegetables, lean proteins, and healthy fats to help support your overall health and weight loss goals.

- Don't overdo it: It can be tempting to overindulge during your eating window, but it's important to remember that intermittent fasting is not an excuse to eat unhealthy foods in excess. Stick to a balanced diet to support your weight loss efforts.

- Be patient: Weight loss is not always a linear process, and it may take some time to see results with intermittent fasting. Be patient and consistent with your fasting practice and you will likely see progress over time.

- Find a method that works for you: As mentioned, there are several different methods of intermittent fasting to choose from. It's important to find a method that works for you and fits into your lifestyle. If one method isn't working for you, don't be afraid to experiment andtry a different approach.

- Don't skip meals: It's important to eat regular, balanced meals during your eating windowto ensure that you're getting all of the nutrients your body needs. Skipping meals can lead to feelings of hunger and may lead to overeating later on.

- Get enough sleep: Adequate sleep is crucial for overall health and weight loss. Aim for 7-9 hours of sleep per night to help support your fasting efforts.

- Stay active: In addition to fasting, it's important to engage in regular physical activity to support weight loss and overall health. Find an exercise routine that you enjoy and try to incorporate it into your weekly routine.

- Don't rely solely on fasting: While intermittent fasting can be a helpful weight loss tool, it should not be the only focus of your weight loss journey. It's important to also focus on a healthy diet and regular physical activity for long-term weight loss success.

- Seek support: If you're having trouble sticking to your fasting routine or if you have any concerns about your health, it's important to seek support from a healthcare professionalor a registered dietitian. They can help you create a plan that works for you and address any concerns you may have.

In conclusion, intermittent fasting can be a powerful tool for weight loss when done responsibly and with the guidance of a healthcare professional. It's important to find a method that works foryou and fits into your lifestyle and to remember that it should be paired with a healthy diet and regular physical activity for long-term success. By following these tips and seeking support whenneeded, you can effectively incorporate intermittent fasting into your weight loss journey and achieve your health goals.

Intermittent Fasting for Women

Chapter 3

Fasting and Fountain of Youth!

I n this chapter, I will explore the relationship between intermittent fasting and youthfulness in women. As we age, it is natural for our bodies to go through changes that can impact our energy levels, metabolism, and overall health. Many people turn to various methods in an effort to slow down the aging process and maintain a youthful appearance.

3.1 Women and fasting

It is a widely held misconception that women should not fast because it is detrimental to their health. While this may be the case for some women, it is not a generalization that can be made for all women. This hypothesis came about because intermittent fasting has the potential to induce a hormonal imbalance in some women if the fasting is not done properly. However, when the right care and precautions are taken, women are able to fast successfully. This led to the development of this theory.

Women are more susceptible to the effects of possible malnutrition than males are since their bodies were anatomically and biologically intended to carry infants. In the event that a woman's body detects that she is about to go hungry, it will react by elevating her levels of the hormones leptin and ghrelin, which are responsible for regulating appetite. Even if a woman is not pregnant at the moment, her body will respond with this hormone reaction in order to safeguard a fetus that is in the process of growing.

Even though it is feasible to ignore the hunger signals from ghrelin and leptin, doing so becomes progressively difficult when the body rebels and begins to create more of these hormones. This is especially true when the body is in a state of starvation. If a woman gives in to her hunger in a manner that is detrimental to her health, such as by overeating or ingesting foods that are detrimental to her health, this might set off a chain reaction of additional hormonal disorders within insulin.

This procedure has the potential to disable the reproductive system as well. If your body believes that it does not have enough food to survive, it may stop the capacity to conceive in order to safeguard a possible pregnancy. Because of this, women who are pregnant or who are attempting to conceive should not fast, and neither should women who are not pregnant.

3.2 The Human Growth Hormone

HGH, also known as human growth hormone, is a hormone that occurs naturally and is created by your pituitary gland. The pituitary gland is a tiny endocrine gland located in the brain that is also responsible for controlling your adrenals and thyroid. When your body produces HGH, the hormone is released into the bloodstream, where it remains until it is converted by the liver into other active growth factors, such as insulin-like growth factor, also known as IGF-1. Every cell in your body can benefit from the growth that these growth factors encourage. When you go without food for an extended period of time, your body responds by producing more growth hormone

(HGH). In point of fact, a number of studies have demonstrated that the levels can rise by as much as five times in comparison to periods when you are not fasting.

The potential of HGH to increase the production of collagen in both the skeletal muscles and the tendons is among the most significant benefits that this hormone provides. Muscles and tendons that contain more collagen result in greater muscle strength, which can improve your physical skills and exercise performance. Muscles and tendons that contain less collagen result in decreased muscle strength. Your resting metabolic rate will increase as a result of having a higher muscle mass.

Even when you are not actively moving about, your body will be able to burn more calories as a result of this. Lipolysis, a physiological process in which fat and triglycerides are broken down andtransformed into free fatty acids, which are then eliminated from the body, is also increased by HGH. This allows for a greater rate of fat loss. A higher rate of lipolysis corresponds to an easierand more rapid process of losing weight.

So what does this have to do with women and youth? Well, these benefits may be particularly relevant for women and youth, as they may be interested in maintaining or improving muscle strength and physical performance, and in losing weight or improving body composition. However, it's important to note that the use of HGH as a performance-enhancing substance or for weight loss is controversial and may have potential side effects, and it should only be used under the supervision of a healthcare professional. It's also important to note that the body naturally produces HGH, and engaging in healthy behaviors such as eating a balanced diet, getting enoughsleep, and exercising regularly can support the body's natural production of HGH and help to promote overall health and well-being.

Chapter 4

Different Types of Fasting and the Best Method forYou to Follow

You're ready to start your voyage of fasting, but before you do, I want to give you some advice onthe kinds of foods you should eat so that the outcomes of the intermittent fast you choose to followare complemented and enhanced to the greatest extent possible. Before I get into what you should eat and what you should avoid eating, I want to offer you some words of encouragement to help you get into the correct frame of mind and clarify your fasting and fasting goals. I'll get tothat in a moment. After that, I look at what you need to know about what foods to consume, whatfoods to avoid, and why you need to know it in language that's easy to understand.

4.1 Before starting your fasting plan

4.1.1 Your goal when fasting should be to deplete any glucose stores youhave.

Follow a proper fasting regimen in order to reach the optimal state of fasting, which takes place when the body has used up all of its glucose (blood sugar) reserves. After you have used up all of your glycogen stores, also known as the carbohydrates that are stored in your muscles and liver, your body will enter a state known as ketosis, which is the state of burning fat for fuel. At that point, the metabolic switch takes place, and alternate sources of energy, such as fat, are ableto be digested and utilized as a fuel in the form of ketones

During your fast, you must abstain from consuming any significant sources of calories so that youdo not throw off your body's natural processes and prevent yourself from entering a ketotic condition. Your pancreas will secrete insulin whenever you take calories, regardless of whether those calories come from carbohydrates, fat, or protein; this will cause the metabolic switch to beturned off. Insulin is necessary for the metabolism of protein, just as it is for carbohydrates and lipids.

4.1.2 Consume foods that are good for you; this is the

purpose of your meal.

When it is time to feast, choose a diet that is good for your health and is based on plants from theMediterranean region.

Do not listen to the useless advice to consume a diet that is high in protein and low incarbohydrates. These diets have been shown to increase the risk of developing diseases such as diabetes, colon cancer, and cardiovascular disease if they are followed for an extended periodof time. Follow the recommendations of nutrition professionals who have spent years researchingthe best way to eat in order to stay healthy. Diets centered on plants and whole foods, such as those found in the Mediterranean, produced the best benefits.

4.1.3 What You Are Allowed to Consume During Your Period of Fasting

The end of your fasting window has arrived; what should you do now? If you've done your homework, you should be able to grab the beverage of your choice and start chugging it down.In the following sections, I will explain what kinds of foods you are allowed to take throughout yourfasting windows to speed up your progress.

4.1.3.1 Consuming liquids to help you get through your intermittent fast

There are a lot of different liquids that you may put in your mouth to assist satisfy your appetite while also maintaining your health and keeping you hydrated. You might be shocked to learn that artificial sweeteners are permitted throughout your periods of fasting. This is a highly contentiousissue; nonetheless, the findings of the scientific community cannot be disputed. According to the findings of a new meta-analysis that was published in the European Journal of Clinical Nutrition,consuming non-nutritive sweeteners does not cause an increase in the level of glucose in the blood.

Additionally, there is a school of thought that maintains that artificial sweeteners do not satisfy the body's biological need for sugar in the same way as sugar does, which may result in an increase in the amount of food consumed. This hasn't been proven. In point of fact, studies have shown that switching from sugar to artificial sweeteners can aid in weight loss for people.

Sweeteners like Splenda and stevia are common choices because they have almost no calories.Although there is no scientific evidence to suggest that either one is dangerous, it would appear that stevia, which is produced from plants as opposed to being manufactured in a laboratory, is connected with the fewest problems.

4.1.3.2 What You Are Allowed to Consume While You Are Fasting

• Do sip plain old water (and lots of it). Don't add any flavorings that are high in calories.

- Do drink unflavored, calorie-free sparkling water, seltzer water, mineral water, and zero-calorie-flavored drinks.

- Avoid drinking calorie-containing fluids at all costs.

- Consume your coffee black, regardless matter whether it's caffeinated or decaffeinated. The information is continued in the following section.

- Do not add anything other than a sugar substitute that is calorie-free (if so desired).

- Consume only tea that has been brewed, whether it be herbal or regular.

- Do not add anything other than a sugar substitute that is calorie-free (if so desired). Tea must be brewed, and there should not be any sugar added. Include a sweetener that is devoid of calories (if desired).

- Do take diet drinks. Avoid drinking any canned or bottled beverages that contain calories,including sodas.

- Chew gum that is free of both calories and sugar (if you so wish).

- Chewing ordinary gum or mints shouldn't be done.

Consume these sweeteners, which are permitted on the Most Popular Intermittent Fasting Plans meal lists, but do so in moderation. It is not easy to go without food for an extended amount of time, therefore if you find that using artificial sweeteners helps you get through your fasting periods, you should not hesitate to do so.

4.1.3.3 Having a passion for black coffee

Since dark chocolate was deemed the new health food, black coffee has emerged as the most significant development in the realm of nutrition to take place in recent times. The question of whether or not coffee is good for one's health has been a source of contention for a very long time. You have reason to celebrate if you are someone who enjoys coffee, as recent research has shown that coffee is, in fact, a healthy beverage to consume. To reap the full benefits of thisfood's positive impact on your health, you must, of course, exercise portion control and avoid consuming any additives.

What about the stimulant caffeine that is found in coffee? To put things into perspective for you: The amount of caffeine that is often found in a cup of brewed coffee that is a standard 8 ounces is between 80 and 135 mg, whereas the amount of caffeine that is typically found in a cup of green tea that is a standard 8 ounces is only about 15 mg. There are 336 mg of caffeine in a handful of coffee espresso beans that have been wrapped in dark chocolate. This amounts to 28beans. A cup of brewed tea containing 6 ounces contains approximately the same amount of caffeine as four roasted espresso beans with 24 mg.

4.1.3.4 A look at the potential positive effects of coffee on one's health

Recent studies have established a link between coffee and a wide variety of positive effects on one's health, and experts agree that it is safe to consume up to eight 8-ounce cups of coffee eachday. Several of the findings are as follows:

People who drank between one and eight cups of coffee per day had a longer life expectancy than those who didn't drink any coffee at all, according to the findings of a huge study that was recently published in the journal JAMA and which involved the participation of half a million people. It should be noted that this was an observational study, which simply demonstrates a correlationand does not prove a cause-and-effect relationship. Researchers presenting their findings at a conference hosted by the American Heart Association have shown a positive correlation between consuming coffee and lowering one's chance of developing cardiovascular diseases such as heart disease and stroke.

The researchers looked at information that was collected as part of the decades-long FraminghamHeart Study. This study looked at the relationship between people's diets and the health of their cardiovascular systems. In comparison to people who did not drink coffee, those who did drink coffee had a lower chance of getting heart failure by 7 percent and of having a stroke by 8 percentfor each additional cup of coffee that they drank each week. This was found in relation to the consumption of coffee.

Regular coffee users had a significantly lower risk of acquiring type 2 diabetes, according to the findings of a review study that was recently published in the journal Dialectology and Metabolic Syndrome. This conclusion was reached after the researcher's analyzed data from previous research. Coffee consumption of a moderate amount (equivalent to or less than four cups of coffee per day)has been found to be the dose most strongly connected with a reduced risk of developing type 2diabetes.

Researchers have hypothesized that the high quantity of antioxidants found in coffee may increase insulin sensitivity, which may, in turn, contribute to a reduced chance of developing type2 diabetes. The findings of a study that was published in the British Medical Journal found that men who drink two to three cups of coffee a day have a 4 percent lower risk of developing gallstones than those men who don't drink coffee regularly, and men who drink four or more cupsof coffee a day have a 45 percent lower risk of developing gallstones.

Consumption of coffee has been shown to play a role in reducing the risk of neurodegenerative illnesses such as Alzheimer's disease and Parkinson's disease, according to some findings from certds According to the findings of a study that was recently published in the journal Frontiers in Neuroscience, drinking coffee, particularly coffee with a dark roast can prevent the formation of amyloid plaques, which are harmful protein aggregates that are a signature feature of dementia.

Additional research has found that drinking coffee is associated with a number of other health advantages, including:

A recent study that was published in the Journal of Nutrition revealed that women who drink twoor three cups of coffee per day have lower whole body and abdominal fat than those who drink less and discovered that women who drink less had higher levels of fat throughout their bodies. The minimal amount of calories that are included in coffee is another reason why nutritionists encourage drinking it. In addition, coffee has been shown to improve one's mood, a phenomenonthat is likely attributable to the presence of caffeine in coffee. Caffeine is an alkaloid that is derivedfrom plants and can be found in a wide variety of foods and beverages, including coffee, tea, and chocolate, as well as certain kinds of soda, energy drinks, and other sorts of sports items. Caffeineis the most widely used illicit substance in the United States, despite the fact that the law considersit to be a drug.

By inhibiting the activity of a certain brain chemical (adenosine) while at the same time stimulatingthe creation of another molecule, caffeine can make you feel more alert and improve your mood (serotonin). For instance, consuming chocolate causes a substantial boost in serotonin, which isa hormone associated with a positive mood. Caffeine acts as a stimulant for the central nervous system, which causes an increase in heart rate and blood pressure. It also stimulates the adrenalglands to produce more adrenaline, which in turn provides a boost in energy. The way an individual reacts to caffeine is unique to them, and many people build up a tolerance to its effects over time. As a result, they are not impacted by the potential negative side effects of caffeine, which include jitteriness, nervousness, upset stomach, and an inability to sleep.

Boost for antioxidants: A cup of coffee can do more for you than just wake you up in the morning;it can also have other benefits. In point of fact, coffee beans are the best source of antioxidants for those living in the United States. Antioxidants remove potentially harmful free radicals from the body, which assists the immune system in its fight against the disease. Free radicals are dangerous by-products of metabolism that act in a manner similar to that of terrorists. They leadto the development of a wide variety of chronic diseases, including cancer and heart disease. Increasing the number of antioxidants you consume will assist your body in neutralizing the effects of free radicals and warding off disease. Coffee's high antioxidant content will help reduce inflammation and lower the likelihood that you may get an illness.

4.1.3.5 Observing how coffee can assist you in remaining successful throughout your fast.

During your fasts, drinking black coffee can be beneficial and is an extremely helpful tool for youto have. Your appetite will be squelched by black coffee. Increases the amount of energy that you feel you have:

Helps you get through the fast more easily.

When you drink your coffee black, you are able to appreciate the coffee's true flavor, and once you become accustomed to drinking it this way, there is no going back! I strongly suggest that you investigate the myriad of flavor nuances that coffee has to offer. You're going to find out thatcoffee is loaded with one-of-a-kind flavors that can titillate your senses. Because cream and sugarmask flavors are to the point where you don't even realize they are present, a true coffee connoisseurshould only consume black coffee.

Not to mention the fact that drinking coffee black is exceptionally convenient. You can go practically anywhere and get a cup of black coffee without having to worry about whether or not they serve your preferred flavored additions.

For those who choose to engage in intermittent fasting, drinking coffee is by no means required.If you can't have coffee, try tea, particularly black or green tea, which has been shown to have health benefits similar to those of coffee.

4.1.3.6 Not everyone should consume caffeine.

Consuming caffeine can have a variety of effects on various people, and individuals' tolerance levels to the substance can vary widely. People who are sensitive to caffeine may experience unpleasant side effects even from consuming small doses of the stimulant, including nausea, anxiety, restlessness, and insomnia. If you are sensitive to caffeine, you should switch to decaffeinated coffee so that you can reap the benefits of the antioxidant increase without experiencing the jitters that caffeine causes.

4.1.4 Feasting

During the times when you are allowed to indulge in feasting, it is up to you to decide what kindsof meals you will consume.

I would advise you to go with the more strategic combination, which I will refer to as the " intermittent fasting strategy." If you give yourself healthy food, your body will reward youwith good results. You are well on your way to creating a powerful disease-prevention and anti-aging lifestyle by combining the Mediterranean diet, which is known for its emphasis on plant-based foods, with the style of intermittent fasting that you have chosen for yourself. You can't argue with the fact that the Mediterranean Diet is good for your health, and the fact that the cuisineis so delicious is just a significant added plus. In this section, I will discuss the different kinds of food that you ought to consume during the eating windows of your intermittent fasting plan in order to get the most out of it.

4.1.4.1 Knowing what foods to consume: Some quick tips

You will have more energy and see better results from your workout if you make it a goal to fill your meals with food that is high in nutrients and has a controlled portion size (including slow, complex carbs to prevent blood sugar swings during your fast). This is the kind of eating that youwould do if you followed a plant-based diet.

During your eating window, here are some short guidelines to follow:

Snack on nutritious foods such as a handful of nuts, some fresh fruit with non-fat Greek yogurt, an apple with some peanut butter, or fresh veggies dipped in hummus.

Avoid consuming calories through liquids unless you're having a glass of red wine with your dinner. It is easy to consume massive numbers of calories in a short length of time if you drink sugary soft drinks, juices, or iced teas, especially if you gulp them down in one sitting. Whole grains, lean proteins (mainly plant proteins), lots of vegetables with deep colors, extra virgin oliveoil, and meals that are seasoned with salt substitutes like citrus, garlic, kinds of vinegar, fresh herbs, andspices should make up the foundation of a well-balanced diet.

The combination of foods that are abundant in nutrients will supply you with the energy you requireto maximize the positive effects of your journey toward intermittent fasting.

Why consuming a diet based primarily on plants is a wise choice

The prevention of cardiovascular illnesses, which are the leading cause of death in both men and women in the United States, is greatly aided by dietary choices. The things that are normally consumed when that are whole-food, plant-based, and low in processed foods have an abundance of disease-fighting compounds that are provided by Mother Nature.

To mention a few of these compounds, they are:

Polyphenols: Polyphenols are compounds found in plants that, when ingested on a regular basis, can improve the health of the digestive tract and the brain, in addition to providing protection against cardiovascular disease, type 2 diabetes, and even certain malignancies. Plant foods, such as fruits, vegetables, herbs, spices, tea, dark chocolate, and wine, are excellent sources of polyphenols due to their natural abundance. They are powerful antioxidants and have the ability to both reduce inflammation, which is the primary factor in the development of many chronic diseases, as well as neutralize potentially harmful free radicals.

Resveratrol is yet another nutraceutical that may be discovered in the meals that come from the plant world and is worthy of a specific investigation. Because red wine is made from dark red and purple grapes, which are rich in resveratrol, red wine contains the highest concentration of this compound. However, blueberries, peanuts, and pistachios also contain resveratrol. It is widely known that the heart-protecting activities of resveratrol and its ability to lower blood pressure are due to the antioxidant capabilities of resveratrol.

In addition, resveratrol causes a rise in adiponectin concentrations, which is significant because adiponectin is a hormone that has a beneficial anti-inflammatory impact.

Carotenoids are plant pigments that give many fruits and vegetables their vibrant red, yellow, and orange colors. Carotenoids are responsible for the coloration of plants. Carrots, tomatoes, pumpkins, papayas, nectarines, and seaweed are all good sources of them, although seaweed has the highest content overall. Their antioxidant and anti-inflammatory properties are likely responsible for the positive impact they have on lowering the risk of having a heart attack.

4.1.5 Keto and intermittent fasting?

Because the timing of your meals is the primary focus of intermittent fasting rather than the foods themselves, you are responsible for selecting the kind of diet to follow in conjunction with your fasting schedule. It is my recommendation that you steer clear of selecting the Ketogenic Diet as your combined eating plan of choice. This recommendation may come across as confusing to you given the amount of internet buzz that promotes the ostensible ideal combination of keto and fasting. People who mix the ketogenic diet and intermittent fasting do so in order to further stimulate the ketosis process in their bodies. In this section, I go into greater detail on why you shouldn't follow the Keto Diet and intermittent fasting together, as well as how the list of permittedand prohibited items doesn't line up properly.

4.1.5.1 Having an understanding of the reasons why the Ketogenic Diet and intermittentfasting do not go together

The following are some of the reasons why the Ketogenic diet is not a good option for those whowish to engage in intermittent fasting:

Dieters who follow the ketogenic diet frequently experience weight loss but in an unhealthy manner. The Keto Diet is associated with an increased risk of cardiovascular disease due to thediet's low fiber content and significant reliance on saturated fat. According to research that was published in the journal Nutrients, many adherents have a diet that is heavy on meat and includesan excessive amount of red and processed meats. This type of diet has been shown to increasethe risk of dying from cardiovascular disease. In addition, the Ketogenic Diet can be harmful to the microbes that live in your gut, which are an essential component of your metabolic health. A prolonged state of ketosis is hazardous to one's health. Ignore the hype, and don't give in to the temptation of eating in order to promote additional ketosis (the process that takes place in your body when it doesn't have enough carbohydrates to burn for energy). Instead, fat is burned, which results in the production of substances known as ketones, which the body can then use for fuel.

While the ketogenic diet also puts your body into ketosis, it does so in an unhealthy way because it is overly restrictive, does not allow for certain foods that are extremely nutritious, and is difficult to stick to. Intermittent fasting, on the other hand, puts your body into ketosis for short time periods before feeding it the nutrients it needs to prevent disease. Intermittent fasting is safe and effective.

It is not the diet that puts your body into ketosis; rather, it is the fasting phase. The fact that you have complete control over when and what you eat is, without a doubt, one of the most appealing aspects of the intermittent fasting method.

Choose your eating plan intelligently, though, if you want to maximize the positive effects that your journey into intermittent fasting will have on your health and fitness. The Keto Diet does not provide enough nutrients. The Keto Diet is just an outdated, extremely high-fat, high- high-protein, and -low carbohydrate eating plan that has been repackaged as a modern, highly appealing, and tremendously popular fad eating plan. This eating plan is rich in fat and low in carbohydrates. The foods that are being marketed have an exceptionally high concentration of unhealthy fats and protein from animals.

In point of fact, the diet necessitates that approximately 80% of your daily caloric intake come from fat, the majority of which is deemed to be unhealthy fat. It is unknown whether or not adopting this diet for an extended period of time will have a negative impact on the health of the heart. Thediet plan excludes several items that are the primary sources of antioxidants, which can help prevent disease and stop the progression of free radical damage.

4.1.5.2 What's wrong with ketogenic diets: What you ought not to consume and what youreally ought to eat

The Keto Diet is notorious for its excessive consumption of items that are known to contribute tothe development of disease, such as red meat and other fatty, processed, and salty meals. This diet recommends a large number of foods, the vast majority of which do not provide your body with the nutrients it requires to preserve and improve its health.

The following is a list of items that are frequently recommended on the Keto Diet but that you should not consume and alternatives for healthier living:

Coconut oil contains a high percentage of saturated fatty acids, which are known to block arteries.It is recommended that you make your primary fat source extra-virgin olive oil (EVOO) and that you occasionally substitute canola oil for coconut oil. Meats that have been processed and red meats both have a high dietary cholesterol and saturated fat content. Consuming red and processed meats are linked to an increased risk of dying prematurely and developing colon cancer.Make lean fish and plant proteins the primary sources of protein in your diet. » Cheeses that contain their natural moisture and rinds are known as full-fat cheeses. These cheeses tend to be high in dietary cholesterol and saturated fats. Make the switch to cheeses with decreased fat content and use a tasty, full-fat cheese in very small amounts as a garnish instead. Full-fat dairy

products, such as whole milk, include a significant amount of dietary cholesterol and saturated fats. Make the switch to milk without fat or to an alternative made from plants.

The Ketogenic Diet prohibits you from eating the following foods, although they are thevery foods that the diet encourages you to consume:

Legumes, which include beans, peas, lentils, and peanuts, are packed with a ton of nutrients; in fact, eating a diet high in lentils has been linked to a longer life. Increasing one's diet of beans, which are rich in antioxidants, has been shown in a number of studies to reduce one's risk of obesity, diabetes, and overall mortality, in addition to fostering improved energy and lower bodyweight.

The high magnesium content of beans helps to strengthen bones, which is an additional benefit of eating beans. Magnesium is a mineral that plays a role in maintaining healthy bone metabolism. The consumption of beans, particularly dark beans, has been shown to significantly improve heart health. Beans do not contain any cholesterol, which, in addition to their high fiber, potassium, folate, and vitamin B6 levels, and their phytonutrient density, all contribute to heart health. Because of this one-of-a-kind fiber's ability to reduce overall cholesterol levels in the blood and notably levels of the harmful LDL cholesterol, it is true that "beans, beans, healthy for your heart!"

In addition to this, beans are an excellent source of nutrition for the powerful microorganisms that reside in our digestive tract and play an important role in the prevention of disease. Cereal grains, which include rice, pasta, and oatmeal: It is absurd to exclude certain grains, which are necessary for maintaining life, even though they should be entire grains. You are going to need the fiber and a considerable amount of nutrients that is provided by these carbohydrates to help maintain and promote a long and healthy life

Goods from the dairy industry that are low in fat:

Dairy products provide the majority of people with a healthy dose of calcium and protein. They should be consumed in the fat-free version in order to rid the body of the arterial-clogging saturated fat that is contained in whole dairy foods. The vast majority of fruits, with the exception of lemons, limes, tomatoes, and very small percentages of berries: It is absurd to omit any fruit. One significant factor that may be contributing to the current epidemic of obesity is the fact that around 90 percent of individuals do not consume enough fruits and vegetables for optimal health.

The majority of alcoholic beverages, including wine:

Drinking red wine in moderation has been shown to reduce the risk of heart disease and is an essential component of the Mediterranean Diet. Vegetables high in starch, such as corn, potatoes, and peas, are a type of carbohydrate known as a "slow carb." Slow carbs are plant foods that are high in fiber and, as a result, take longer to digest and cause a slower rise in blood sugar. Starchy vegetables, such as corn, potatoes, and peas, should be included in a healthy diet, and in particular, an intermittent fasting program. Be sure to incorporate some of these in your daily intake.

The best strategy to improve health and longevity is to follow a diet that is plant-based and high in whole foods, such as the Mediterranean Diet. This type of diet is also the most beneficial addition to a lifestyle that includes intermittent fasting. The intermittent fasting, rather than the diet, is what initiates metabolic switching and cellular stress resistance. These are the primary triggers for the myriad health benefits that this way of life offers. Bear in mind that breaking a fast for the first time can be challenging.

4.2 The 16:8 Time-restricted Intermittent Fasting Plan

A growing number of people are turning to intermittent fasting as a method for improving not only their weight but also their general health. The time-restricted plan is the most common variant (and also the most straightforward) of the intermittent tent fast. This type of fasting, often known as the eating-window diet, is one of my personal favorites. You are in control of when and for how long your window of opportunity to eat is open.

When you practice time-restricted intermittent fasting, you restrict the amount of time you spend eating and not eating to a predetermined number of hours each day. This period of time is referredto as the "eating window."

The 16:8 intermittent fast is the most frequent time-restricted pattern. This is where you eat all ofyour meals for the day in an 8-hour period, and you can eat whenever you want during this window. Your fasting period lasts for the following 16 hours, during which time you do not ingest any calories (only calorie-free beverages and lots of water). You follow the same routine each and every day.

This chapter focuses on the 16:8 intermittent fasting plan and includes guidance on how to followit. Although there are several variations to the time-restricted intermittent fasting plan, this chapter is dedicated to discussing the 16:8 plan.

The majority of people consume some form of nutrition from the moment they awaken till the moment they go to sleep. When you engage in the practice of time-restricted eating, you are, in essence, restricting the total number of hours that you spend eating each day. It's easier than traditional dieting because you don't have to count calories or limit your favorite foods when you follow this time-restricted eating approach to intermittent fasting, which is why it's become so popular. When you switch from the traditional style of eating (three meals and snacks) to this time-restricted eating approach, you'll naturally eat fewer calories and lose weight. People who allow themselves to consume all of their usual calories within their eating window are more likely to failat this form of fasting than those who do not do this.

Your daily "eating window" refers to the period of time during which you are permitted to consumefood while adhering to the time-restricted intermittent fasting method of dieting. You decide on the time frame and hours that are going to be most conducive to your way of life and the most sustainable. This plan does not give you permission to binge eat anything and everything you want during the allotted time for eating. Creating a calorie deficit on a daily basis is still the primaryobjective for weight loss and fat burning. This means eating fewer calories on a daily basis than you were accustomed to eating.

Other intermittent meal plans, such as 17:7, 18:6, and 20:4 are choices you have in addition to the 16:8 plan, which is probably the most common and easiest plan for you to begin with. However, you can choose to follow one of these other plans. In this chapter, I will focus exclusivelyon the 16:8 intermittent fasting plan, explain how it operates, and help you determine if this is thetype of intermittent fasting that you want to begin practicing right away.

4.2.1 Putting the time-restricted 16:8 strategy to the test

The 16:8 intermittent fasting diet is the easiest one for you to begin with because it is so simple and requires so little work from you. On the 16:8 plan, you limit your eating to a window of eight hours, such as from 10 a.m. to 6 p.m., and then you go without food from 6 p.m. to 10 a.m. the following day. Martin Berkhan, the author of The Leangains Method, is credited with being the first person to bring widespread attention to the 16:8 intermittent fast.

With the time-restricted intermittent fasting regimen known as 16:8, you pick the 8 hours of the day during which you consume all of your daily calories, and you stick to that pattern every day. The 8-hour eating window is the most forgiving of all the many types of intermittent fasting because, in comparison to other time-restricted eating patterns, the 8-hour time frame allows for a greater degree of flexibility in terms of what you can consume within the eating window. Additionally, you may quickly map out the eating window hours that are most convenient for you during the day.

If you want to lose weight, you should make sure that the number of hours you spend eating is less than the number of hours you normally give yourself permission for. To put it another way, if you are accustomed to eating over a period of ten hours, you will want to make sure that you cut your eating window down to considerably less than ten hours (the lower, the better). If you find that the 16:8 method works well for you or if you want to push yourself further, you can shorten the amount of time you spend eating each day to anywhere from four to twelve hours, which equates to fasting for sixteen to twenty hours.

4.1.6 Understanding the simplicity behind the 16:8 plan

Because it is a more moderate time-restricted feeding protocol than any of the other types of intermittent fasting, the 16:8 diet has gained a lot of popularity in recent years. In point of fact, as compared to other intermittent fasting plans, this food pattern is very close to being identical to anormal eating pattern. This eating pattern translates into a routine of skipping breakfast each dayand not eating after dinner on a daily basis, and many people find themselves inadvertently adhering to this eating pattern. Because people normally sleep for approximately half of the 16 hours that they need to fast, the 16:8 approach is very popular for newcomers.

To clarify, persons who follow time-restricted intermittent fasts lose weight because the method forces them to eat during shorter windows of time than they were accustomed to, which in turn causes them to consume fewer calories on a daily basis. It is hypothesized that if you limit the amount of time that can be spent eating, you will consume less food overall than you did in the past. If you skip meals but then make up for it by overeating at the times you are allowed to eat, you will not be able to lose weight.

Consider the following scenario with a person who adheres to the time-restricted intermittent fasting protocol of 16:8: John's objectives are to preserve his health and fitness and reduce the amount of body fat that he carries. Before John, age 45, started doing intermittent fasting, he would typically take his first meal around eight in the morning and continue eating (and drinking)until approximately ten in the evening. As a result, he restricted himself to eating only during a window of 14 hours each day.

John made the decision to begin a time-restricted intermittent fast, and as a result, he shortenedthe length of his eating window (the number of hours in which he ingested food on a daily basis)to a period of eight hours. He realized that the most convenient way for him to eat was to restricthimself to eating just during a window of eight hours (repeating the same eight-hour window eachand every day), which meant that he had to eliminate two of his meals or snacks.

John reorganized his routine such that he would begin eating at midday and continue until 8:00 p.m., which was a time frame that was most accommodating to both his job and family obligations.In addition to that, he kept up with his daily aerobic routine by performing it first thing in the morning, practiced breathing exercises for relaxation and rhythmic breathing for five minutes immediately before lunch, and crammed in a strength-training program twice a week right after work. After following this plan for a period of six months, John was able to shed five pounds of body fat, bring his fasting blood sugar level down to less than 100 mg/dl, bring his LDL cholesterol numbers down, and boost his HDL cholesterol levels. In addition, he raised his HDL cholesterol numbers.

4.2.2 Shedding the fat while preserving the muscle mass

Keeping up with your regular strength-training routines while adhering to a time-restricted fasting diet is the most effective approach to ensure that you just lose fat and not the muscle mass that you have worked so diligently to acquire. Also, before beginning any kind of workout regimen, especially one that involves exercising while also intermittently fasting, you should make sure to acquire clearance from your primary care physician.

If you are a physically fit and muscular individual who is following a time-restricted intermittent fast in order to gain the health benefits, maintain your lean body mass, and lose some body fat, then I have some good news for you: some sound scientific data supports the effectiveness of this strategy.

Regrettably, there has not been a sufficient amount of research conducted on time-restricted eating to be able to determine the duration of the eating window is optimal. On the other hand, an article published in the esteemed New England Journal of Medicine in December 2019 evaluatedthe most recent scientific research on intermittent fasting and the accompanying health benefits that can be attained from doing so.

The authors recommended that medical professionals prescribe intermittent fasting as an early intervention strategy for patients who were already suffering from a variety of chronic conditions or were at risk for developing such conditions, particularly those conditions that were linked to excessive eating and leading a sedentary lifestyle. To be more specific, they recommend a transition period of four months in order to successfully achieve the objective of achieving an 18:6time-restricted intermittent fasting pattern. The following is the prescription for it:

Eating window of 10 hours, 5 days per week for the first month • Eating window of 8 hours, 5 daysper week for the second month • Eating window of 6 hours, 5 days per week for the third month.The fourth month will have a six-hour eating window, seven days a week. According to the findingsof the researchers, a metabolic switch from glucose-based energy to fat-based ketone energy can be effectively triggered by restricting eating to a 6-hour window once every 18 hours while simultaneously fasting for 18 hours.

This metabolic trigger is associated with an increase in resilience to stress as well as a larger potential for longevity. In addition, the scientists believe that following the 18:6 intermittent fastingplan can increase a person's resilience to diseases such as cancer and obesity, which is yet another health benefit of the strategy.

The 16:8 diet and the conventional diet were both tested on a total of thirty-four muscular and physically healthy men, with the average age of the participants being thirty years old. Both groupsof guys kept up with their typical routines of strength training with weights. During the 8-week period of the experiment, the 16:8 subjects ate three meals per day at 1 p.m., 4 p.m., and 8 p.m.,and then fasted for the remaining 16 hours out of every 24-hour period.

These meals were spaced out so that they consumed 100 percent of their daily calorie needs (thenumber of calories needed to maintain their current body weight). The people in the control groupsplit their daily calorie intake into three meals, which they ate at 8:00 am, 1:00 pm, and 8:00 pm. This was done so that they could keep their existing body weight.

What were the results?

Both groups kept their levels of muscle mass constant throughout the study. Only the 16:8 group,however, saw significant improvements in both health and body composition. Those who participated in intermittent fasting shed a sizeable amount of body fat (around 2.5 pounds) and saw a reduction in the amount of inflammation in their systems. In addition, only the group who practiced intermittent fasting saw a reduction in the amount of sugar and insulin in their blood.A large rise in adiponectin levels was also observed in the group that had been fasting, which is important to note.

Only adipocytes, often known as fat cells, are capable of producing and secreting the hormone known as adiponectin. The hormone adiponectin is responsible for regulating both the fat and sugar metabolisms in the body.

In humans, insulin resistance and type 2 diabetes are both associated with significantly reduced levels of the hormone adiponectin found in the blood. The ability of intermittent fasting to increaseinsulin sensitivity is responsible for the observed increase in adiponectin levels as well as the decrease in insulin levels seen in the 16:8 intermittent fasting group. Increased insulin sensitivityis a well-known effect of increased adiponectin levels. Additionally, because of its anti-inflammatory properties, adiponectin contributed to the reduction in inflammatory markers that were observed in the fasting group.

One of the most important aspects of the time-restricted fasting technique that was used in the study was that the total daily calorie intake was kept the same for both groups. The only thing thatwas changed for the fasting group was the amount of time that passed between meals. Simply the order in which food was consumed has an effect on body composition and health indices. A useful training method for athletes who do resistance training is time-restricted intermittent fasting,which consists of 16 hours of fasting and 8 hours of eating.

This helps athletes enhance health-related biomarkers, reduce fat mass, and at the very least retain muscle mass. The cutting phase of a bodybuilder's training, also known as the maintenancephase, has the objective of keeping the same amount of muscle mass while decreasing the amount of fat mass. During this phase, a bodybuilder could use a routine like this one.

4.2.3 Do not turn your eating session into a binge

After settling on a particular time each day to consume food, the next question is what kinds of foods to consume and how frequently. That is dependent upon the goals that you have. If you aretrying to lose weight by engaging in intermittent fasting, you need to make sure that your eating window does not turn into an all-out binge session during which you consume an excessive amount of food. If your goal is to lose weight, the fundamental reason that intermittent fasting is effective is that it causes you to consume fewer calories on a daily basis. You will probably not lose any weight at all and may even put on some if you binge eat and consume enormous amounts of food while you are allowed to eat during your eating windows.

4.2.4 An Analysis of the Most Commonly Practiced Variations ofIntermittent Fasting

When beginning a program of intermittent fasting, it is not uncommon for one to first experience feelings of hunger as well as irritability, sometimes known as "hungry." You've probably had this sensation before: you're hungry, and your appetite is only becoming stronger with each passing minute.

Because of your hunger, you are becoming increasingly unpleasant to be around; you are becoming agitated, impatient, and angry. You are beyond hungry now! Realize that you have

complete command over these sensations. The good news is that they will typically disappear within two weeks to a month as your body and brain become adjusted to this new way of living.

While you are fasting, it is important to drink plenty of beverages that do not contain calories, suchas water, black coffee, and tea. During the times when you are allowed to eat, you should focus on eating foods that are high in nutrients. If you do this, it will take the edge off of your hunger andassist prevent you from being irritated as a result of being hungry.

4.3 The Warrior Intermittent Fasting Plan

When you hear the word "warrior," you may immediately think of a Roman gladiator with his well-oiled and well-sculpted rippling muscles bulging from under his scant armor. You may also picturea daring warrior battling lions by hand in the Coliseum.

It would be a mistake to use the use of this word to describe a certain method of intermittent fasting to infer that only adhering to this method of fasting will magically transform you into a fierce warrior.

That doesn't mean that you can't get bigger and leaner if you follow this diet, though. This chaptertakes a look at the Warrior approach to intermittent fasting and provides you with all the information you require to get started.

The Warrior intermittent fasting plan is another type of time-restricted fasting that is also often known as the 20:4 intermittent fast. This kind of time-restricted intermittent fasting is far more stringent than others because the eating window is only four hours long each day. You are permitted to consume more than one meal within your allotted eating window. The Warrior plan is neither the most straightforward method of performing intermittent fasting, nor does it allow forany customizations to be made to the method. If you deviate from the 20:4 protocol, the Warrior intermittent fasting strategy that you are following will no longer apply to you.

The Warrior intermittent fast consists of not eating or drinking anything from the time you wake up until the time you eat again in the evening. This means that you will be fasting for a total of 20 hours. If you want to lose weight, you have to make sure that during your four-hour feasting periodyou don't consume too many calories; otherwise, you'll put on weight instead of losing it. You have the great freedom to eat whatever you want, but for the benefit of your general health, you should make an effort to make sure that the foods you choose to eat are well-balanced and includea lot of nutrients.

4.3.1 The original warrior diet origins and weaknesses

Ori Hofmekler, a former member of the Israeli Special Forces who later switched to the field of health and fitness, is credited with being the one who first brought the Warrior Diet into the mainstream. Individuals are directed by Hofmekler in his best-selling book, The Warrior Diet, which was initially released in 2002, to strive for actually "feasting" during the 4-hour window. They are encouraged to eat 80 to 90 percent of their daily calorie intake within this time period.

During the 20-hour fast, he also permits the consumption of limited quantities of food and snacks, including particular fruits, juices, vegetables, eggs, and dairy products.

The concept behind the Warrior Diet eventually gave rise to the One Meal a Day (OMAD) Diet. The one-meal-a-day diet (OMAD) is a straightforward eating plan in which participants consume only one meal per day, at whichever time of day they regularly eat dinner.

The Warrior Diet consists primarily of an extended period of fasting interspersed with brief periods of eating. The ancient Romans had the belief that eating just one meal per day was optimal for one's health, which is how this eating pattern became associated with the Roman gladiator soldiers. The ancient Romans held the belief that eating more than one meal in a single sitting was an act of gluttony. Enlisting in the Warrior Intermittent Fasting Plan intermittent fasting regimen in which participants are allowed to consume only one meal per day, which can consist of anything they like and is typically consumed in the evening.

The one major difference between OMAD and other time-restricted intermittent fasting plans is that rather than restricting your eating for the standard window of time, which is typically 16 hours(or 20 hours in the case of the Warrior plan), you restrict your eating for a whopping 23 hours (including the time you spend asleep).

4.3.2 Drawbacks of the Warrior Intermittent Fasting Plan

The following are some of the primary advantages and disadvantages of following the Warrior intermittent strategy:

If you want to follow the Warrior intermittent fasting strategy, you have to make sure that you provide your body with all of the nutrition it needs during the 4-hour eating window that you provide yourself each day.

Maintaining the Warrior intermittent fast as prescribed is an excellent method for cultivating discipline. The plan may be challenging for someone who is just starting out with intermittent fasting. It's not easy to go from eating three meals a day to not eating for 20 hours straight. You may eat less. People who follow this strategy frequently report feeling full more quickly and havingless of a desire to consume excessive amounts of food. Consuming fewer calories will lead to weight loss.

If you're an endurance athlete, the Warrior Diet probably isn't the greatest plan for you to follow. It is not possible to meet the exceptionally high caloric needs of these athletes within such a limited time for eating since it is too tough.

You might become less preoccupied with food. People who follow this approach frequently reporthaving fewer thoughts about food and not experiencing feelings of deprivation as a result.

It's possible that your social life will suffer if you commit to a full 20-hour fast and do it every day.

4.3.3 Incorporating Physical Activity into Your Warrior Intermittent Diet

During your Warrior intermittent fast, you can and should still get some physical activity. Weight training is an essential component of any fitness program that aims to increase lean body mass while simultaneously reducing overall body fat. Make it a point to perform your sets of resistance training at the time of day when you are allowed to eat, while you should perform your cardio workwhile you are fasting.

Before beginning any kind of workout regimen, especially one that involves exercising while alsointermittently fasting, you should make sure to acquire clearance from your primary care physician.

4.3.4 Investigating the dietary practices of actual warriors

The Game Changers, a contentious documentary released on Netflix in 2018 concerning the relationship between a plant-based diet, protein, and strength, has been the talk of the weight room as of late. The movie has both increased the popularity of plant-based diets and received agreat deal of negative feedback.

After suffering an injury, elite Special Forces trainer and winner of "The Ultimate Fighter" James Wilks begins researching and implementing a plant-based eating strategy. The documentary, which was executive produced by James Cameron, Arnold Schwarzenegger, and Jackie Chan, follows James Wilks' journey through this process. As a matter of fact, he attributes his improved athletic performance to the new diet that he has been following.

The documentary weaves together ground-breaking scientific research with personal anecdotesfrom Wilks detailing his struggles and eventual victories. The movie stars some of the athletes that are considered to be the most powerful, fastest, and toughest on the entire planet. The voyage of Wilks dispels outmoded illusions about food, such as the debate between plant and animal sources of protein, which not only have an impact on human performance but also on thewellbeing of the earth.

The documentary focuses on a new study that conducted an analysis of the ancient bones of gladiators that were excavated from the graves of 22 gladiators who were buried in the Roman town of Ephesus approximately 1,800 years ago (now Turkey). The analysis of these men's bonesindicated that their diets consisted primarily of wheat, barley, and beans; hence, they were giventhe name "Barley Men."

In addition, ancient Roman records that date back 2,000 years suggest that gladiators followed a particular diet known as gladiatorial Saginaw. This diet consisted mostly of grains and legumes including wheat, barley, and beans. In some modern accounts of gladiator life, the combatants are referred to in a derogatory manner as hordearii, which literally translates as "barley men." Theterm "hordearii" comes from the fact that gladiators were most likely fed grain of worse quality than the general population. The lower quality of diet is a direct result of the fact that the majority of Roman gladiators were recruited from among prisoners of war, slaves, and condemned criminals.

4.4 The Alternate Day Intermittent Fasting Plan

You have a number of options available to you when it comes to the timing of your fasts when you practice intermittent fasting. Investigating each of the available plans can assist you in selecting the one that is most suitable for your unique way of life. While some of the diets are significantly more challenging to adhere to than others, the majority of the diets are rather straightforward.

One other choice is the alternate-day intermittent fasting, which is also known as the 4:3 plan. Of all the diets, this one has the greatest amount of research to back up its claims of being both effective and safe.

4.4.1 An Explanation of the Numerous Variations of the Intermittent andAlternate-Day Fasting Plans

Because you abstain from eating for extended stretches of time during strict alternate day intermittent fasting, this is one of the most rigorous forms of dietary restriction. You start out eatingnormally, but then skip meals for a few days in a row. In other words, you abstain from eating anddrinking for one day, and then you eat what you want something the following day, then you haveto fast the following day, and so on. In other words, during the week you take meals on four daysand fast on three days that are not consecutive.

There are numerous different variations of the alternate-day intermittent fasting pattern. Alternate-day intermittent fasting regimens can take place in a variety of different methods, some of whichare listed in the following list:

On your fast days, you don't eat anything or almost nothing at all, but on your feast days, you caneat as much as you want. On your fasting days, you reduce the amount of food you eat by a thirdto a half, but on your feasting days, you give yourself permission to eat more than your usual foodintake.

This is what some people refer to as "calorie cycling." Because you fast entirely once a week, onMondays, Wednesdays, and Fridays, the total duration of your intermittent fast is three days. Thisvariation is common because weekdays provide you little time to sit down to a meal with your loved ones or close friends.

Even though some Alternate Day fasting schedules only permit calorie-free drinks on fasting days,others allow small amounts of food (typically a maximum of 25 percent of your total daily calories) on fasting days. This can be confusing for people who are trying to lose weight because they thinkthey are only allowed to consume drinks.

4.1.7 A Scientific Breakdown of the Alternate-Day Intermittent Fasting DietPlan

Because I'm a scientist and I enjoy looking at the data, the Alternate-Day Intermittent Fasting planis one of my faves among the several intermittent fasting strategies. It should come as no surprise that there is a wealth of credible scientific information available on the practice of fasting every other day and the attendant remarkable health advantages.

For instance, the results of a randomized clinical trial, which is considered to be the "gold standard" of scientific research that prove a cause and effect relationship, were published in the journal Cell Metabolism. This trial studied the effects of alternate-day intermittent fasting on the body. The findings of the largest study of its kind, which examined the effects of intermittent fastingusing the stringent alternate-day method in healthy persons, revealed a wide range of positive health consequences. The individuals cycled through periods of consuming no calories for 36 hours followed by unrestricted eating for 12 hours.

Researchers from Austria chose sixty participants at random to take part in a study that lasted forfour weeks. All of the participants were of a healthy weight and ranged in age from 35 to 65. The researchers randomized the participants to receive either an Alternate Day or a Continuous Daytreatment. Participants were randomly assigned to either a fasting group or a control group; participants in the latter group were allowed to consume as much food as they desired.

The following findings were found in the group that participated in intermittent fasting:

Even on days when they were not fasting, the group had proof that there was a consistent level of ketones in their blood. It has been demonstrated that an excess of ketones is beneficial to one'shealth in a variety of ways. The group had lower levels of a blood marker called soluble intercellular adhesion molecule-1, which is linked to age-associated illness and inflammation. Triiodothyronine, a hormone produced by the thyroid, was found in reduced quantities among thisgroup, although the thyroid gland continued to operate normally.

There is a correlation between having low amounts of this hormone and having a longer lifespanin humans. The levels of LDL cholesterol and triglycerides in the group had dropped significantly. The group had a reduction in both weight and total body fat (a loss of 9 percent of total body fat,with a particular emphasis on the elimination of dangerous abdominal fat).

On the days that they were supposed to be fasting, these intermittent fasters restricted themselves to drinking only water and resumed their normal levels of exercise.

All of the participants in this study were physically active people in good health, ranging in age from young to middle-aged. Before beginning any type of intermittent fast, you are need to obtain permission from your doctor if you have any preexisting medical ailments or issues.

4.4.2 Advantages from Following an Alternate-Day

Intermittent Fasting Plan

Another study looked at the intermittent fasting regimen known as Alternate Day and found that it has a number of health advantages. An associate professor of nutrition at the University of Illinois named Dr. Krista Varady calls the intermittent fasting strategy known as Alternate Day the Every Other Day Diet. This approach is also known as the Up-Day, Down-Day plan. She is the author of a book as well as a number other solidly crafted studies. A day of restricted eating, during which participants take only 25 percent of the calories necessary for their body, is followed by a day of unrestricted eating, during which they are allowed to consume as many calories as they choose.

Varady included both normal weight and overweight participants in his randomized clinical experiment that lasted for a period of twelve weeks and was published in the Nutrition Journal. The compelling health benefits of the Alternate Day intermittent fast were apparent after a period of 12 weeks of following the regimen. The participants experienced significant weight loss.

At the conclusion of the experiment, participants had lost 6 percent of their body weight, which is equivalent to 11 pounds. There was no change in muscle mass, but there was a 7.7-pound drop in body fat. Additionally, from pre-treatment to post-treatment, there was an increase in both dietary satisfaction and sensations of fullness. Demonstrated favorable shifts in risk factors for coronary heart disease. After a period of 12 weeks, there was a discernible decline in the contentof triglycerides of twenty percent.

In addition, the size of the LDL particles rose after therapy. LDL is the "bad" cholesterol, and a larger LDL particle size indicates better health. Felt less inflammation in their bodies. There was a discernible reduction of the amounts of circulating creative protein (CRP). The CRP protein isa marker of inflammation throughout the body. This protein is produced by the liver. Shown enhanced sensitivity to insulin. An increase in adiponectin, which is a protein hormone that acts as an insulin sensitizer in addition to having anti-diabetic, anti-inflammatory, and anti-atherogenic effects on the body. Intermittent fasting on alternate days has been the subject of a large numberof further scientific studies, all of which have shown positive health effects. The following are someexamples of these:

A study that was conducted in 2013 and published in the Nutrition Journal discovered that participants who followed this intermittent fast protocol for a period of 12 weeks had a loss of roughly 8 pounds of body fat. If middle-aged spread is a problem for you, another recent study found that participants aged 50 to 59 years obtained higher weight loss with alternate-day intermittent fasting compared to people of other age groups.

4.4.3 A First-Hand Account of Implementing the Alternate-Day IntermittentFasting Plan

Diseases of the heart are the primary cause of death on a global scale. Alternate day intermittentfasting helps reduce the risk of heart disease in many different ways. However, the benefits of this form of fasting could be maximized by combining it with a healthy Mediterranean lifestyle, which has been shown to improve cardiovascular health.

Increased insulin sensitivity while maintaining a healthy blood sugar level. When the body is unable to create enough insulin or when it is unable to use the insulin that it does make in an effective manner, high blood sugar levels result (referred to as insulin resistance). Diabetes is a condition that can be brought on by consistently high blood sugar levels. Studies have indicated that a type of intermittent fasting known as "alternate day fasting" can help reduce fasting blood sugar levels by lowering blood insulin levels and boosting insulin sensitivity. Autophagy, the process that recycles unneeded, damaged, and possibly hazardous cell components, was boosted.

Autophagy is the term for the process. Lengthened one's life span (in animals). In animal tests, itwas found that drastically lowering the total number of calories consumed, which may be accomplished by following the alternate-day fasting protocol, considerably increased the length of their longevity.

4.4.4 Incorporating Physical Activity Into Your Cycle of Alternating Days ofFasting

During your regimen of alternate-day intermittent fasting, you can and should continue to engagein physical activity. During your time spent planning out your alternate day intermittent fasting routine, you should give some thought to when and how you want to fit in the various sorts of workouts you do.

You might be wondering why you would want to incorporate physical activity into your routine of intermittent fasting on alternate days. The solution is straightforward: so that you can accelerate the process of losing weight! A study that was published in the journal Obesity revealed that participants increased their rate of weight loss by using cardio. Sixty overweight people were randomly assigned to one of four groups:

- Exercise alone

- Exercise + cardiac exercise

- No diet or exercise

- Exercise alone and Alternate day fasting alone (diet)

When compared to each individual strategy, fat was burned at least twice as efficiently by the people who followed a combination of the Alternate Day intermittent fasting regimen and cardiac exercise. The researchers also demonstrated that the combination caused improved changes inbody composition (a large decrease of body fat while maintaining muscle mass) and reduced indications of heart disease risk in comparison to the separate therapies.

Before beginning any kind of workout regimen, especially one that involves exercising while alsointermittently fasting, you should make sure to acquire clearance from your primary care physician.

4.5 The 5:2 Intermittent Fasting Plan

The 5:2 fasting regimen, commonly known as the most well-liked kinds of intermittent fasting, is a type of alternating periods of eating and fasting. It's possible that the intermittent fasting diet is even the most well-known one out there. Continue reading to find out if this intermission The FastDiet, often known as the tent fast, is one of the diets that may be adapted to suit the preferencesand requirements of each individual participant.

4.5.1 Providing Clarification on the 5:2 Plan for Intermittent Fasting

On five days of the week, you eat as you normally would, and on the other two days of the week,you restrict your caloric intake to between 500 and 600 per day. This is called the 5:2 intermittent fasting strategy. You should drink only water for one to two days out of the week that are not consecutive. In addition, it is recommended that you should consume 500 calories if you are a woman either in one meal or spread out over the course of the day; this should account for a quarter of your daily calorie needs.

On the other five or six days of the week, you are free to consume as many calories as you want, whenever you want, and you do not even need to give calorie restriction a second thought. You are free to select any two days of the week for your fast, as long as there is at least one day in between them on which you do not restrict your food intake.

4.5.2 Understanding the 5:2 method of intermittent fasting

It is possible that some individuals will find it simpler to adhere to this strategy as opposed to, for example, the Alternate Day Intermittent Fast. It may be appealing to a big group of individuals to have to restrict their food intake only one or two days each week, and then not have to worry about what they are going to eat for the remaining five or six days of the week.

Michael Mosley, a British broadcaster, is credited with popularizing the 5:2 strategy for intermittent fasting. It is said that he developed the 5:2 intermittent fast after being diagnosed with type 2 diabetes and wanting to reverse the condition naturally rather than relying on medication. Michael Mosley Presents Horizon: Eat, Fast, and Live Longer was a BBC documentary that Mosley shot in 2012 and it quickly became quite famous. After that, in 2013, he released the book The Fast Diet.

4.5.3 Investigating the Scientific Basis Behind the 5:2 Rotational FastingPlan

In addition to a substantial body of scientific support, the intermittent fasting regimen known as the 5:2 ratio is one of my personal favorites. Mark Mattson, PhD, a neurologist at Johns Hopkins, has spent the past quarter of a century researching intermittent fasting and the mechanics underlying it. He has published a number of controlled human studies that study the effects of a variety of intermittent fasting regimens, the most common of which was the 5:2 intermittent fastingdiet.

The results of his study demonstrated the following:

His study of one hundred overweight women demonstrated that those on the 5:2 intermittent fasting diet lost the same amount of weight as women who restricted calories, but they did betteron measures of insulin sensitivity and reduced belly fat than those in the calorie-reduction group.

A battery of cognitive tests showed that two hundred twenty adults who were healthy and not fat and who followed the 5:2 intermittent fasting protocol for two years exhibited signs of better memory. Based on these findings, it appears that intermittent fasting may offer neuro-protective therapies that can help ward off dementia and neurodegeneration.

It may take some time for your body to adapt to the intermittent fasting regimen you are following. The early negative effects of intermittent fasting are not uncommon, and they can include feelings of hunger as well as anger. The good news is that they usually disappear within two weeks to a month, as the body and brain become acclimated to the new eating routine.

4.5.4 Implementing the 5:2 Rotational Intermittent Fasting Plan

According to a website hosted by Johns Hopkins University, which provides a summary of an article published in The New England Journal of Medicine, the following are some of the things that intermittent fasting on a 5:2 ratio is believed to be able to improve:

• Improvements in cardiovascular health Intermittent fasting has been shown to improve cardiovascular health in a number of ways, including lower resting heart rate, lower bloodpressure, and improvements in a number of other heart-related parameters.

• Brain performance: a number of studies have shown that intermittent fasting can increasecognitive abilities. According to a number of studies, adults who engage in intermittent fasting experience improvements in their verbal recall. One study indicates significant fatloss in active guys while preserving their muscle mass, which is beneficial to both their athletic performance and their body composition.

• Wound healing: Studies show that intermittent fasting reduces the amount of tissue damage that occurs during surgery and improves the overall results of the procedure. » Blood sugar level: Numerous studies have shown that intermittent fasting results in significant weight loss and normalization of blood glucose.

The 5:2 diet is an additional strategy that can assist your body in entering autophagy, a process characterized by cellular regeneration.

4.5.5 Keeping Active While Following the 5:2 Diet Intermittent Fast

Any type of intermittent fast, including the 5:2 intermittent fast, is enhanced by the addition of physical activity. When you do cardio while you are fasting, you receive the added benefit of enhanced insulin sensitivity as well as fat reduction, which is a winning combination. This is why doing cardio while fasting is so advantageous.

Before beginning any kind of workout regimen, especially one that involves exercising while alsointermittently fasting, you should make sure to acquire clearance from your primary care physician.

4.6 The Eat-Stop-Eat Intermittent Fasting Plan

There are many different ways in which you can include an intermittent fasting regimen into yourdaily routine. One technique that is known as the Eat-Stop-Eat intermittent fast is garnering more and more attention these days. This chapter covers all you need to know about this type of strategy, including how to apply it, whether or not it is beneficial for weight reduction, and any potential negatives you need to consider before jumping in headfirst.

4.6.1 Taking a look at the Eat-Stop-Eat Intermittent Fasting Plan

When you follow the Eat-Stop-Eat intermittent fasting regimen, which is also known as the 24- hour fast, you select one or two days of the week that are not consecutive during which you totallyabstain from eating for a full 24-hour period. During this time, you are considered to be fasting. During the 24-hour fast, you are not allowed to ingest any food other than beverages that are calorie-free. Therefore, your objective is to go without eating for a full day at a time without any breaks in between.

The eat-stop-eat intermittent fasting regimens are something to think about. Making your own calendar is a good idea. You are able to consume something on each of the seven days of the week, in spite of the fact that doing so may appear paradoxical. You could, for instance, eat normally up until six o'clock on a Tuesday, and then abstain from food until six o'clock on the following Wednesday, after which you would resume your normal eating schedule.

According to Brad Pilon, the Canadian author who popularized this intermittent fasting plan in hisbook Eat Stop Eat, if you can't make it the full 24 hours, 20 hours will also work (although if you did that, technically it would be the 20:4 plan, which is also called the Warrior plan). You are freeto consume anything you want for five or six days out of every week.

This strategy is perfect for continuing a daily fitness program or beginning a new one if you are only going to be fasting once per week. Just remember to acquire clearance from your primary care provider before beginning any sort of workout plan.

In the following parts, I will analyze the benefits and drawbacks of the Eat-Stop-Eat diet and look at some research that demonstrates its usefulness.

4.6.2 Comparing the advantages and disadvantages

The Eat-Stop-Eat intermittent fast is similar to the 5:2 strategy in that adhering to it has both positive and negative aspects to it. Some of the benefits and drawbacks are outlined:

• Because you just abstain from food for one day at a time, it is more adaptable and lessdifficult to follow in comparison to other, more severe fasting programs.

• It can be challenging to abstain from food for the full period of twenty-four hours.

• People who have some days of the week when they are

extremely busy or sociable and other days of the week when they are less social and it would be simpler for them to fast will find that this method works well for them.

• After the beginning of the eating period, there is a risk of eating more than necessary.

• Numerous positive effects on one's health, including but not limited to reduced body fat, increased insulin sensitivity, decreased levels of hormones associated with appetite, and preservation of muscle mass.

• It's possible that you won't be able to maintain a fast of 24 hours once or twice a week over the long run.

• Does not impose any limits on food intake or any other types of restrictions. The possibilityof unfavorable repercussions on one's health.

• Does not encourage calorie tracking or weighing meals in any way. It is challenging to take part in social activities that entail food, such as going out to eat with friends or attending parties.

4.6.3 Getting Started with the Eat-Stop-Eat Intermittent Fasting Plan

Keep in mind that regardless of which intermittent fasting strategy you choose, the following are some advice I have for you to follow in order to achieve the results you desire:

Maintaining a consistent practice, eating mindfully, and consuming a plant-based, whole foods, Mediterranean-style diet while feasting are all important parts of a healthy lifestyle. Do not consider the days when you are not fasting to be an open invitation to a food festival.

4.6.4 Taking into consideration what the research reveals

The 5:2 diet, Alternate Day fasting, and the 16:8 forms of intermittent fasting have all been the focus of a significant amount of research in the medical and scientific communities. Although it is not referred to as "Eat-Stop-Eat" in the scientific literature, there is a significant amount of research on what is termed weekly one-day fasting or periodic 24-hour fasting. This is essentiallythe same plan as the Eat-Stop-Eat version of intermittent fasting, but it is not called "Eat-Stop- Eat" in the scientific literature.

Researchers at the Intermountain Medical Center in Salt Lake City, Utah, looked at the impact ofa water-only fast lasting for twenty-four hours on aspects of health other than weight loss. The purpose of the study was to gain an understanding of the physiological shifts that take place in the body during a period of fasting lasting for twenty-four hours. The clinical trial was known as the FEELGOOD trial, and it was carried out over the course of a two-day participation period witha total of thirty healthy individuals who were randomly assigned to either the fasting group or theeating group. Multiple health markers were obtained from both groups, and their combined data was examined. The following results were obtained from the subjects who participated in the fasting group:

The level of human growth hormone (HGH), which is produced by the pituitary gland in the brainand is significantly increased when a person is fasting, was shown to be much higher.

HGH helps the body burn fat, in addition to building muscular mass and speeding up the metabolism. During the period of fasting, both the total number of red blood cells and the hemoglobin level increased. The body encourages regeneration of the entire circulatory system when it is subjected to fasting cycles, which is beneficial to the health of the cardiovascular system.

Triglycerides and total cholesterol both went down when fasting, whereas high-density lipoprotein cholesterol and total cholesterol both went up. Fasting had an opposite effect on HDL cholesterol.It is very protective against heart and vascular disease to have a higher level of the beneficial HDL cholesterol and a lower level of the harmful lipids known as triglycerides. Trimethylamine N-oxide: The amount of a substance known as trimethylamine N-oxide that is found in the blood drops dramatically when a person fasts (TMAO). Human gut microbiota are the source of the biomarker known as TMAO, which is associated with an increased risk of cardiovascular disease.

When people consume food, the bacteria in their gastrointestinal tracts break it down and produce a chemical known as trimethylamine (TMA). The TMA is subsequently converted into the molecule known as TMAO by the liver. The problem with TMAO is that studies have shown that high levels link to an increased risk for clot-related events such as heart attacks and strokes. This is a significant drawback of TMAO.

In addition, research conducted by scientists has demonstrated that elevated TMAO levels in the blood are linked to an increased risk of passing away at an earlier age. Therefore, intermittent fasting has the beneficial effect of altering the micro biome in a way that moves it away from a composition that is conducive to cardiovascular disease.

Fasting also dramatically reduced blood levels of the amino acids proline and tyrosine. Lower levels of circulating proline and tyrosine are associated with lower rates of insulin resistance, improved cognitive performance, and reduced levels of depression. The level of urea in the fasting group's blood was found to be substantially lower than in the other groups.

You are in charge, you decide what should be done, and you devise the plan that will serve your needs in the most efficient manner. Stick to the recommended eating plan to get the most out of both worlds and get ready to take pleasure in this incredible journey toward improved health and wellness. In addition, make sure to consult with your medical professional before beginning any new fitness routine.

Chapter 5

Autophagy

Autophagy is a normal physiological process that is involved in the cleaning out of old or destroyedcompounds in the body. It does this by consuming and digesting them. The term "autophagy" literally means "self-eating," which can be a little unsettling to hear because of the way it sounds.It comes from the Greek terms autos, which means "self," and phagein, which means "to feed." Together, these phrases give us the English word "autophagy." After a group of researchers noticed an increase in lysosomes in liver cells in response to injections of glucagon, the hormonethat acts in opposition to insulin, Christian de Duve, a scientist who had previously won the NobelPrize, came up with the term autophagy to describe this process. Autophagy is the part of the cell that is responsible for breaking down and destroying other compounds.

The process of autophagy is critically important to the body's ability to sustain homeostasis or a steady and healthy internal environment. Proteins and organelles, which are small, specialized structures found in each of your body's cells, are continually in the process of becomingdysfunctional or dying in your body. These dead tissues, if allowed to build in the body, can leadto the loss of cells, contribute to poor tissue and/or organ function, and even cause cancer if the accumulation is allowed to continue. During the process of autophagy, the body identifies damaged cellular components and proteins that are no longer being utilized. These broken-down components are transported to the lysosomes, where they are degraded and eventually eliminated from the body. Because of this procedure, they won't be able to cause any harm.

This process has been referred to as an inborn recycling program by Dr. Colin Champ, a radiation oncologist who holds board certification and is an assistant professor at the University of Pittsburgh Medical Center. He believes that the process of autophagy makes your body more effective by removing any malfunctioning portions, putting an end to any metabolic dysfunction (such as obesity and diabetes), and preventing malignant (and potentially cancerous) growths from occurring.

5.1 What happens if there is no autophagy?

If autophagy is not "turned on," then dead proteins will continue to be present in the body and willbegin to build up. These dead proteins are linked to the development of chronic disorders, the most notable of which are cancer and Alzheimer's disease. Plaques are a characteristic feature of Alzheimer's disease, which is defined by the accumulation of one or two of these proteins— amyloid beta or tau protein—which accumulate in the brain and contribute to the formation of plaques.

In addition, there is evidence suggesting that autophagy may have a role in both the reduction of chronic inflammation and the enhancement of natural immunity. According to research conducted on the topic, persons who are unable to induce autophagy have a propensity to be larger in size,to sleep more frequently, to have higher cholesterol levels, and to have diminished cognitive function.

Because it involves denying the body of specific foods for a predetermined amount of time, fastingis one of the most efficient strategies to induce autophagy in both the body and the brain. This isbecause fasting switches the process on. After eating causes an increase in insulin, which causesglucagon, the hormone that works in opposition to insulin, to decrease. On the other hand, glucagon levels rise when insulin levels fall (which happens after a period of time during which there is no food). Glucagon levels rise during fasting, which encourages the process of autophagy.

After a period of abstaining from food, the body experiences a large rise in the number of autophagosomes, which are the organelles responsible for the disposal of cellular waste. After a period of fasting, the number of autophagosomes in the body might increase by as much as 300percent, according to the findings of certain research.

5.2 Other Methods That Can Help You Boost Autophagy

You may also kick on this process by exercising and by following a ketogenic diet. Fasting is themost efficient approach to promote autophagy, but you can also do it by exercising and by fasting. Because of this, a lot of people who fast also elect to follow a ketogenic diet as well because it has a double effect on cleaning out the cells in the body.

The ketogenic diet is similar to fasting in that it tricks the body into thinking it is lacking food, whichresults in the same metabolic alterations. This helps to induce autophagy. When you dramatically reduce the amount of carbohydrates you eat, it compels your body to switch to using fat as its primary source of energy. Maintaining insulin levels at low levels and glucagon levels at high levels is essential for initiating the process of autophagy.

Regular exercise has been demonstrated to kill malignant cells and is therefore an efficient approach to promote autophagy, which is one of the most effective ways to stimulate autophagy.One study that was published in the journal Autophagy indicated that the rate of autophagy considerably increased after running on a treadmill for thirty minutes and continues to grow up toan overall total of eighty minutes of exercise, at which point it begins to level out. When exercisingat a high intensity, the effect might be observed to a greater degree.

Chapter 6

How to Begin and Deal with Food Lust

While intermittent fasting can be beneficial for both men and women, it can be difficult to start andstick to the routine. One common challenge is dealing with food cravings and the constant desireto eat, also known as "food lust." In this chapter, I will discuss how to begin intermittent fasting and how to effectively deal with food lust while following the intermittent fasting routine.

To start intermittent fasting, it's important to choose a fasting schedule that works for you. Thereare several options to choose from, including the 16/8 method (fasting for 16 hours and eating during an 8-hour window), the 5:2 diet (eating normally for 5 days and restricting calories to 500-600 on the other 2 days), and the alternate-day fasting method (fasting every other day). If you'renew to intermittent fasting, it may be helpful to gradually work up to your chosen fasting schedule.

For example, if you're starting with the 16/8 method, you could begin by fasting for 12 hours andgradually increasing the fasting window over time. During your eating window, it's important to eat a balanced diet and focus on whole, unprocessed foods to ensure you're getting all the nutrientsyour body needs. It's also important to stay hydrated, especially if you're going for longer periodswithout food.

Dealing with food lust while following an intermittent fasting routine can be challenging, but thereare strategies you can use to manage it. One way to deal with food lust is to eat satisfying meals during your eating window. Choose high-protein, high-fiber foods that will keep you feeling full and satisfied for longer periods of time. It's also helpful to practice mindful eating by paying attention to your food and eating slowly, savoring each bite.

This can help you become more aware of your hunger and fullness cues and can help you avoidovereating. When you're feeling the urge to eat, try finding a non-food related activity to do instead, like going for a walk or reading a book. Staying busy can also help distract you from foodcravings and can make the time pass more quickly during your fasting window. Finally, it's important not to be too hard on yourself if you have cravings or slip up and eat more than you hadplanned. It takes time to adjust to a new way of eating, so be kind to yourself and try to get back on track with your next meal or snack.

In addition to the strategies mentioned above, there are a few other things you can try to help manage food lust while following an intermittent fasting routine. One option is to eat smaller, more frequent meals during your eating window. This can help keep your blood sugar levels stable and can reduce the risk of overeating. Another option is to incorporate healthy fats into your diet, as they can help keep you feeling full and satisfied. Healthy fats include avocado, olive oil, nuts, and seeds. It's also helpful to plan ahead and have healthy snacks on hand for when you're feeling hungry during your fasting window. Some good options include nuts, hard-boiled eggs, or a piece of fruit.

It's also important to be mindful of your emotions when it comes to food lust. Sometimes, our desire to eat is driven by emotions rather than actual hunger. If you find yourself constantly craving

food, it may be helpful to take a moment to pause and consider what's driving those cravings. Are you feeling stressed, anxious, or bored? Finding healthy ways to cope with these emotions, like going for a walk or practicing relaxation techniques, can help reduce the urge to eat constantly.

Finally, it's important to remember that intermittent fasting is not a quick fix or a one-size-fits-all solution. It's a long-term approach to eating that requires patience, commitment, and self-awareness. If you're having trouble sticking to your intermittent fasting routine or if you're experiencing negative side effects, it may be helpful to consult with a healthcare professional or a registered dietitian. They can provide guidance and support to help you find the approach to eating that works best for you.

Chapter 7

Meal plan

A "one size fits all" approach is not appropriate when discussing nutrition. A diet that is specifically designed for you will be the most effective way to eat, just as a custom-tailored garment would fit you best. Having said that, there are certain general nutrition concepts that you may use to determine which foods work for you and which ones don't by comparing them to each other.

Although abstaining from food for a considerable amount of time is the primary objective of fasting, you should still make an effort to have nutritious meals during the times that you are allowed to break your fast and eat. This will guarantee that your nutritional requirements are met and that you are providing your body with all of the nutrients it requires to remain healthy and full of energy.

7.1 Figuring Out Which Diet Is Best for You to Follow

Keep in mind that the actual definition of diet is "the type of food a person habitually eats," and that is how you should interpret the term here. Although the term diet is commonly associated with some type of food restriction, the real definition of diet is "the type of food a person habitually eats." If you want to gain the most benefits from intermittent fasting, it is important to choose a diet that is high in foods that have not been processed and are rich in nutrients. However, there is no required diet that you must follow in order to do so.

There are various diets that are commonly used in conjunction with intermittent fasting, but you shouldn't get caught up in the dogma around these diets. You don't have to stick to a diet plan to the letter if it doesn't work for you. For instance, if you choose to adhere to the guidelines of the Paleo diet but later learn that your body functions optimally when it consumes brown rice, you are free to include it in your diet. If an item doesn't fit a particular diet's category, that doesn't mean you have to cut it out of your diet completely. Eat with your intuition in order to determine the strategy that will serve you best.

7.2 Ketogenic Diet

Alongside intermittent fasting, the ketogenic diet has become one of the most common dietary trends in recent years. People who enjoy intermittent fasting are likely to gravitate toward this diet since the two approaches complement each other nicely: when taken together, they'll swiftly throw you into a chronic state of ketosis. This diet is also a good choice for people who want to lose weight (a physiological state in which your body burns fat for energy instead of carbohydrates).

When you are adhering to a ketogenic diet, you will get the majority of your daily calories from fat, and you will drastically limit the amount of carbohydrates that you consume. A ketogenic diet, in contrast to other diets, requires you to carefully monitor the quantities of fat, carbohydrates, and protein that you consume on a daily basis.

The following is an example of a typical ketogenic diet's breakdown of macronutrients:

• Fat accounts for 60–75 percent of the total calories

• 15–30% of total calories should come from protein

• 5–10% of total calories derived from carbohydrate sources

7.3 Low-Carb Diet

Restricting the number of carbs you consume on a daily basis is a key component of both a ketogenic diet and a low-carbohydrate diet. On the other hand, a standard low-carb diet does notcontain nearly as much fat as a ketogenic diet does and permits a protein consumption that is more modest. Many low-carb diets recommend beginning with a very low-carbohydrate consumption for a short period of time, typically around two weeks, during which time you cut outpractically all meals that contain carbohydrates, with the exception of low-carb vegetables.

During this initial phase of the program, you will experience a large loss of water weight. After these two weeks, you will transition to a program that is more sustainable and will allow you to incorporate nutritious sources of carbs, such as additional veggies, some fruits, and gluten-free whole grains. Standard low-carbohydrate diets have as their primary objectives the reduction of insulin and blood sugar levels, as well as the promotion of weight loss.

7.4 Paleo Diet

Another popular method that is often used in conjunction with intermittent fasting is the Paleo Diet.Just like fasting, the Paleo Diet is based on the eating patterns of your ancestors. Consuming just those foods that might have been obtained by foragers and hunters during the time period knownas the Paleolithic is the central tenet of the Paleo diet. This term is, of course, subject to interpretation due to the fact that your Paleolithic ancestors would not have had access to modern conveniences such as jars of almond butter; nonetheless, you get the general concept.

When adhering to a Paleo Diet, the following foods are permitted:

- Meat

- Fish

- Avian and Fowl

- Eggs

- Seeds and nut products

- Fruits

- Non-inflammatory fats (avocado oil, coconut oil, olive oil, ghee)

- Natural sweeteners (raw honey, maple syrup, coconut sugar)

On the other side, you should steer clear of the following:

- Grains (wheat, oats, barley, rye, quinoa, couscous, amaranth, millet, corn)

- Dairy (milk, cheese, ice cream, butter)

- Legumes (soy, peanuts, chickpeas, beans)

- Alcohol

- Sugars and sweeteners, both refined and fake (white sugar, high-fructose corn syrup,sucralose, aspartame)

The question of whether or not corn should be categorized as a vegetable or a grain generates a lot of discussion. Corn is not permitted on the Paleo Diet because, despite its reputation as a vegetable, it is more accurately classified as a whole grain. In addition to this, the majority of thecorn that is cultivated in the United States comes from GMO (genetically modified organism) crops, which are something that proponents of the Paleo Diet aim to stay away from.

7.5 Pegan Diet

Dr. Mark Hyman, who is also the director of the Center for Functional Medicine at the Cleveland Clinic, came up with the idea of the Pegan Diet, which is a relatively recent eating plan. At first glance, the Paleo Diet and a vegan diet appear to be on completely different ends of the spectrum;however, their basic principles are actually very similar. The Pegan diet combines the basic principles of both diets, which seems counterintuitive because the diets appear to be oncompletely different ends of the spectrum.

The Paleo Diet and a vegan diet both stress the importance of selecting complete, unadulteratedfoods that are derived from the earth in an ethical manner. A vegan diet does not include any animal products and places an emphasis on grains, legumes, vegetables, and other plant-basedfoods. On the other hand, the Paleo Diet places an emphasis on meats that have been sourced in an ethical manner, vegetables, healthy fats, and certain fruits, and it does not include any legumes or grains. The Pegan diet is an attempt to integrate the benefits that are associated withtwo different diets into one.

When following the Pegan diet, around 75 percent of your daily consumption should be comprisedof foods derived from plants. Consume a diet that is primarily composed of vegetables, along with some fruits, a small amount of gluten-free grains (such as quinoa, brown rice, and gluten-free oats), and a small amount of legumes (such as lentils). The remaining 25 percent of your daily caloric intake should be composed of high-quality animal proteins (beef that has been grass-fed,chicken that has been pasture-raised, and eggs), as well as nutritious fats such as coconut, olives,and avocados (and their respective oils: coconut oil, olive oil, and avocado oil). Dr. Hyman suggests using meat less as a primary dish and more as an accompaniment to other foods. Stickto a serving size of 2–3 ounces of meat per meal rather than the customary 4–6 ounce portion.

Gluten, dairy products, and certain types of vegetable oils are off limits when following a Pegan diet (canola, sunflower, corn, and soybean). Consumption of sugar, especially in its natural formssuch as honey and maple syrup, should be limited to special occasions only. Even though consuming natural sugars in moderation can provide some health benefits, consuming an excessive amount of them can have a detrimental effect on blood sugar levels, which is something that you want to avoid as much as possible when practicing intermittent fasting.

7.6 Low-FODMAP Diet

Short-chain carbohydrates are referred to as FODMAPs. FODMAP is an acronym that stands for fermentable oligosaccharides, disaccharides, monosaccharides, and polyols. People who are sensitive to their digestive systems may experience stomach discomfort while consuming FODMAPs. Diets low in fermentable oligosaccharides, polyols, and polyol esters (low-FODMAP diets) are often prescribed for people who suffer from irritable bowel syndrome or persistent digestive issues for which there is no known cause If you are following a diet that is low in FODMAPs, you will **avoid** particular groups of carbs, including the following:

- Wheat, rye, legumes, garlic, onions, leeks, asparagus, jicama, fennel, beetroot, andBrussels sprouts are examples of foods that contain oligosaccharides.
- Disaccharides include white sugar, dairy products such as milk and yogurt, as well as softcheeses like cream cheese and cottage cheese.
- Peaches, plums, pears, nectarines, mangoes, watermelons, apples, and honey are examples of foods that contain monosaccharides.
- Polyols: blackberries, avocados, sweet potatoes, cauliflower, snow peas, and mushrooms blackberries, avocados, and

mushrooms

When you are on a diet that is low in FODMAPs, you will refrain from eating any foods that are high in FODMAPs for around one month. After this initial phase of elimination, you will be able to slowly reintroduce one meal that is rich in FODMAPs to evaluate how your body reacts to it. If youdo not experience any digestive discomfort after eating a certain item, it is likely that your body is able to process it. If you do, there is a good chance that you are sensitive to it, and it would be best for you to steer clear of it as much as possible.

7.7 Basic Nutrition Elements

It is not required to restrict oneself to a certain dietary principle, as a matter of course. Experimenting with various food types and determining which foods work for you and which foodsyou should steer clear of can be facilitated through the application of fundamental nutrition principles. These principles include consuming only fresh, whole foods; avoiding processed foodsand sugar; and consuming an abundance of fruits and vegetables.

7.7.1 Grains

The discussion surrounding grains is very lively. It would appear that nutrition specialists, as wellas the general people, are split down the middle regarding the question of whether or not grains are beneficial to one's health. On one side of the argument, it is

Melissa May

suggested that people steer clearof grains, while on the other, it is argued that whole grains are essential due to the amount of fiberand vitamin B that they contain. So, who is in the right here? The short response is that it is not always the case. According to those who advocate avoiding grains, there are three significant drawbacks to consuming grains: lectins, phytates, and gluten.

7.7.2 Lectins

Lectins are a type of protein that can be found in grains as well as legumes. They are known to bind to the membranes of cells. Because they are resistant to heat as well as the digestive enzymes, they are very difficult to digest. They are also quite small. Because of this, they have apropensity to build up inside of your body and then go through your bloodstream in their whole form. When complete proteins enter your bloodstream, your immune system produces antibodies,which indicates that it identifies the protein as a foreign intruder and constructs a defense mechanism to combat it. This happens when the protein enters your bloodstream in its native form. This can, over time, result in a leaky gut as well as an increased sensitivity to lectins.

The production of lectins is an important part of a plant's defense system. They serve the purposeof preventing harmful creatures, insects, and other critters from feeding on the plant and causingits death. Lectins are resistant to digestion, and as a result, they go

114

through the digestive system unaltered. This allows the plant to regrow after the lectins have been eliminated.

7.7.3 Phytates

Compounds known as phytates can be found in higher concentrations in legumes and grains, with lower concentrations in nuts and seeds. Phytates are not inherently harmful to your health; rather, they are frequently referred to as antinutrients due to the fact that they inhibit the absorption of minerals such as calcium, iron, and zinc by binding to these minerals. This puts you at risk for developing mineral deficiencies. It is essential to keep in mind that phytates do not inhibit your body's ability to absorb nutrients over the long term; rather, they merely prevent the absorption of nutrients during the meal in question.

7.7.4 Gluten

When it comes to grains, gluten is, without a doubt, the subject of the most debate. In contrast to the widespread acceptance of celiac disease, which is characterized by an inability to effectively digest gluten, many individuals do not believe in non-celiac gluten sensitivity. However, research suggests that gluten can harm the intestinal lining (and induce symptoms of celiac disease) even in those who do not have the condition.

Researchers at the University of Maryland found that when people consume gluten, their bodiesmanufacture a protein known as zonulin. This discovery was made possible by gluten. Zonulin has a deleterious effect on the gut lining because it loosens the typically highly tight junctions between the cells that line the intestinal tract. When these spaces are established, food and microorganisms are able to enter the bloodstream because they are able to travel through them.When these particles reach the bloodstream, they set off an immunological reaction that is neverstopped once it has begun. This response has the potential to result in inflammation as well as potentially lead to chronic illness. In addition to this, it is the primary contributor to the development of many autoimmune illnesses. This condition is referred to as "leaky gut," and current research indicates that individuals who consume gluten have at least a mild version of it.

7.7.5 A Remark Concerning Wheat

Wheat is one of the most important crops grown anywhere in the globe, and its use in agriculturedates back more than nine thousand years. Because it can be kept in its kernel form for years without spoiling and because it can be processed into such a broad variety of meals, including flour, breads, noodles, and cereals, it is regarded to be an essential component of the food supplyin many countries. The issue with wheat is not the grain itself but rather the changes that have been brought about by current agricultural practices.

Not only does current wheat contain lesser levels of several nutrients than wheat from the past did, but the structure of the plant itself has also been altered as a result of modern milling techniques. The purpose of current methods is to generate a crop that is able to live in the eventthat a disaster strikes. To achieve this goal, big food firms have made the crop resistant to drought,harsh weather, pests, and chemicals. As a direct consequence of this, your body no longer recognizes wheat in the same manner in which it formerly did. As a result, rather than being nourishing, it now causes inflammation and is addicting.

7.7.6 Improving the nutritional value of grains

If you want to eat more grains, there are a few things you can do to help your body digest them better. If you want to include grains in your diet, read on. First, make sure to choose grains that are gluten-free. It is estimated that approximately one percent of the population has celiac disease, and up to thirteen percent of people have non-celiac gluten sensitivity. Some of the symptoms of gluten sensitivity are as follows:

- Gassiness

- Abnormal bowel movements (constipation or diarrhea)

- Abdominal pain

- Pain in the head

- Fatigue

- Skin problems (rashes, psoriasis, eczema, hives, dermatitis)

- Depression

- A decrease of weight for no apparent reason

- Anemia caused by a lack of iron

- A feeling of unease

- Joint or muscle pain

- Autoimmune diseases

- Fog of thought

Brown rice, wild rice, quinoa, buckwheat, millet, teff, and amaranth are some examples of grainsthat do not contain gluten. Even though oats do not contain gluten in their natural state, they are virtually always cross-contaminated with gluten during the processing that is required to make them edible. If you wish to incorporate oats into your diet, you should look for brands that clearlydesignate their products as being gluten-free.

The following step that you can take before consuming your grains is to soak them. By soaking grains, you can help break down the phytates and neutralize the lectins, making the grains easierto digest and increasing the likelihood that you will be able to absorb all of the nutrients containedwithin them. To prepare the grains for soaking, place them in a dish and cover them entirely withwarm water that has been filtered. You need to put one tablespoon of an acidic medium, such aslemon juice or apple cider vinegar, into the bowl for every cup of water that you put into it. This isa need.

For instance, if you need three cups of water to cover your grains, add three tablespoons of lemonjuice to the water, then cover the bowl with a medium that allows air to circulate, such as a cleandish cloth. This will allow the grains to absorb the flavor of the lemon without going bad. The nextstep is to let the grains settle for a full day. After the grains have been allowed to soak for the necessary period of time, you should wash them in ice water and then continue with the procedureas you normally would.

You also have the option of sprouting your own grains or using grains that have already undergone the sprouting process. Many food producers are aware of the positive effects that sprouting grains can have on one's health. As a result, some manufacturers now provide grains that have already been sprouted, which can save the consumer both time and effort. If you can'tlocate grains that have already been sprouted at the grocery shop near you, you can either huntfor them online or sprout them yourself.

It only takes around seven hours of soaking time to break down brown rice, which is significantlyless time than it takes for some of the other gluten-free grains because brown rice has lower phytate levels.

Because you have to wait for the grain to actually break open and develop a sprout before you can begin sprouting, the process takes a lot more time than simply soaking grains. To sprout your own grains, first follow the steps for soaking them, and then transfer the grains after they have been soaked and drained into a glass container. A Mason jar is an excellent choice for this purpose. After placing cheesecloth over the top of the jar, let the grains ferment in the humid environment for anywhere between one and five days. When they are ready, the grains will break open, and you will be able to see a green sprout emerging from the center of each grain. You can keep grains that have sprouted for up to a week in the refrigerator after you refrigerate them.

7.7.7 Dairy

Another commodity that is fraught with debate in the field of nutrition is dairy. You undoubtedly learned about how beneficial milk is for your bones when you were a child. However, contrary to popular belief, drinking milk does not significantly improve bone health. In point of fact, countries with the lowest consumption of milk also have the lowest rates of fractures and osteoporosis. Osteoporosis is a condition in which the bones become brittle and are more prone to breaks and fractures. Countries with the lowest consumption of milk also have the lowest rates of osteoporosis. In addition, the proteins and carbohydrates that are present in milk might be difficult to digest for a lot of people. This is due to the fact that as you get older, your body's natural production of lactase, which is an enzyme necessary for effective digestion of milk, naturally diminishes.

But this doesn't mean you can't drink any dairy at all; rather, it only means that there are some dairy products that are better for you to ingest than others. If you want to incorporate dairy into your diet, it is best to consume dairy that comes from cows that were given grass. Milk, butter, and cheese made from grass-fed cows are typically stocked in the dairy sections of local supermarkets. In contrast to conventional dairy, which is heavier in omega-6 fats, the omega-3 level of grass-fed dairy products is significantly higher.

Omega-6 fatty acids aren't intrinsically unhealthy but consuming too much of them can lead to chronic inflammation, which is a problem that many Americans face. It's also a good idea to consume grass-fed dairy products that have been cultured, such as yogurt and kefir; just make sure to get the plain, full-fat varieties. Sugar can be found in high concentrations in flavored yogurts and kefirs.

Goat's milk products are an excellent alternative for those who choose to steer clear of cow's milkaltogether. Cattle milk produced in modern times has large concentrations of a protein known asA1 casein, which can cause significant inflammation in the body (and cause issues like eczema and acne). On the other hand, goat's milk has a protein in it called A2 casein, which is anti- inflammatory and does not cause swelling. According to studies, those who drank milk with A2 casein had significantly less inflammation and did not have any unfavorable stomach symptoms.

7.8 Meat and poultry products

Because of the amount of saturated fat that it contains, meat is another contentious food productthat has earned a bad reputation over the years. When low-fat diets became increasingly fashionable, eating red meat was considered to be a major no-no. However, since then, sciencehas demonstrated that saturated fat does not have as great of an impact on heart disease as waspreviously thought. In point of fact, certain kinds of saturated fat can be beneficial in warding off heart disease.

Saturated fat was thought to raise cholesterol, which in turn increased the risk of heart disease. However, recent research has shown that while saturated fats can raise the amount of LDL in your blood, it also creates the large, fluffy LDL particles that don't stick to the artery walls. This contradicts the traditional school of thought. Additionally, consumption of saturated fat leads to anincrease in HDL levels, which is an important factor in the prevention of heart disease.

Additionally, meat is one of the best sources of vitamin B12 there is. In point of fact, vitamin B12can only be obtained through the consumption of foods derived from animals. In addition to the other B vitamins, meat is a good source of vitamin D, vitamin E, amino acids, various minerals, and antioxidants.

In light of the aforementioned, it is essential to select high-quality meats that are grass-fed, just as it is with dairy products. The majority of cattle used to produce conventionally raised beef are given GMO grasses, cereals, and even sugar. This causes the cows to gain weight more rapidly,which increases their production, but it also alters the nutritional profile of the meat they produce. Additionally, grass-fed meat has up to five times the amount of omega-3 fatty acids and a considerable reduction in the amount of omega-6 fatty acids found in conventional meat.

You should strive for a ratio of omega-3 fatty acids to omega 6 fatty acids that is equal to one another. This will help keep inflammation at bay. Omega-6 fatty acids are prevalent in many of today's commonly consumed meals, such as refined seed and vegetable oils, conventionally raised beef, and processed vegetable and seed margarines. Consuming an excessive amount of these foods might throw off this ratio, which in turn can cause your body to experience chronic inflammation.

Conjugated linoleic acid, generally known as CLA, is another type of fat that can be found in grass-fed meat. CLA is an antioxidant that has been found to reduce the risk of heart disease, inhibit the formation of malignant tumors, prevent atherosclerosis, lower triglycerides, and lower the chance of acquiring type 2 diabetes. These benefits have been demonstrated via numerous studies. CLA is found in some quantity in all animal diets; however, meat and dairy products derived from cows that were fed grass have up to five hundred percent more CLA than those derived from grain-fed cows.

As is the case with beef, not all forms of fowl are equivalent. There is fowl that is farmed on conventional farms and there is poultry that is raised organically and allowed to roam freely while eating a natural diet. Both types of poultry can be found in grocery stores. Chickens and turkeysare not vegetarians, despite the fact that labels on poultry and eggs will sometimes boast that thebirds were "fed a vegetarian diet." Chickens and turkeys do not consume vegetarian diets. Theyhave a voracious appetite for grubs, ticks, and worms, which is one of the reasons why chicken is considered to be so nutritious. Poultry that has been given access to a natural diet has a greaterconcentration of healthy omega-3 fatty acids, vitamins, and minerals.

When selecting poultry, it is in your best interest to opt for a breed that was both organically andpasture-raised. Talk to the people who grow your food if you can't find it at your neighborhood grocery shop or if you want to avoid breaking the bank to do so. Because these are terms that are moderated by the government, and many smaller farms are unable to afford to pay for the certification process that is required to carry these labels, you may often find high-quality meats at your local farms that aren't labeled pasture raised or organic, but are, by definition, both of these things. You can find this type of meat at your local farms.

7.8.1 About Eggs

Because of the widespread concern regarding cholesterol levels, many people peel their eggs, dispose of the yolks, and consume only the egg whites in their cooking. Although there is proteinin the egg white, the majority of the egg's nutritional value comes from the yolk, which contains things like vitamin A, vitamin D, vitamin E, vitamin K, B vitamins, omega-3 fats, calcium, and

Phosphorus. The egg white is where you'll find the protein. You shouldn't be afraid to consume the entire egg, but you should be selective about the kinds of eggs that you eat.

Eggs have a lot of labels and promises about their nutritional value, but most of them are really marketing ploys. For instance, the phrases "natural" and "farm fresh" typically do not mean anything specific. Other words, such as "cage-free," have a pleasant ring to them, but they can be deceiving. If you hear the word "cage-free," your first thought could be of birds free to fly aroundin the fresh air and sunshine. However, "cage-free" actually only implies that the birds were not confined in any way.

They might have been still be located in a cramped warehouse with very little available space formovement. Organic eggs that have been reared on pasture are considered to be of the highest quality.

Again, chatting to egg farmers in your area is a terrific way to get high-quality eggs that are typically less priced and fresher than the eggs you'll find in grocery stores. Eggs can be foundin most grocery stores.

7.8.2 Seafood

The most notable health benefits associated with seafood come from two specific omega-3 fattyacids: eicosapentaenoic acid (EPA) and docosahexaenoic acid. Seafood is loaded with protein and beneficial vitamins and minerals, but the most notable health benefits associated with seafood come from two specific omega-3 fatty acids: EPA and DHA (DHA). It has been proven that taking in adequate amounts of EPA and DHA on a consistent basis can lower one's chanceof developing cardiovascular disease, cancer, type 2 diabetes, and autoimmune illnesses.

When selecting fish, it is recommended to ingest species that are smaller in size. The flesh of larger fish that are higher up on the food chain has a greater propensity to accumulate higher levels of mercury as well as other heavy metals and poisons.

The following are examples of fish and shellfish that are particularly rich in omega-3s:

• Salmon

• Mackerel

- Trout

- Sardines

- Herring

- Oysters

- Mussels

However, tuna and swordfish are also high in mercury levels despite their abundance of omega-3 fatty acids. Reduce your intake of tuna and swordfish if you choose these options. There is one company, which goes by the name Safe Catch, that sells tuna in cans that are safer and have thelowest levels of mercury imaginable.

In addition to opting for fish that are lower in size but higher in omega-3 fatty acid content, the ideal kind of fish to consume are those that were captured in the wild rather than those that were reared in captivity. Farm fish are fed a diet that is not natural to them, just as animals that are keptspecifically for the purpose of producing conventional meat. Corn and other grains could fall under this category. Because of their artificial diet, fish that are produced in farms tend to have a higherconcentration of omega-6 fatty acids and a lower concentration of omega-3 fatty acids.

According to a study that was published in the Journal of the American Dietetic Association, omega-3 fatty acids could not even be discovered in some farm-raised fish that was sold in grocery shops. This was the conclusion of an examination that was conducted. Farm-raised fishtend to acquire larger levels of poisons and pollutants in their flesh, in addition to the altered quantities of fatty acids that are present in their bodies.

7.9 Fruits and Vegetables

You are aware that eating fruits and vegetables can be beneficial to your health. There is no denying that some fruits have a higher natural sugar content than others; however, when this sugar is paired with the fiber that is found in the fruit, it does not pose an issue for the majority ofpeople. Because fruit juice contains all of the sugar but none of the fiber, consuming an excessiveamount of fruit juice might be problematic; therefore, while eating fruit, it is important to consumeit in its full form and, ideally, with the skin still attached (which contains fiber).

Research has shown that organic produce not only has lower levels of pesticides and herbicidesthan conventional fruit, but it also has higher levels of certain vitamins and minerals. This is a significant advantage over conventionally grown produce. Utilizing the Environmental Working Group's list of the Dirty Dozen can help you decide which fruits and vegetables are most importantto buy organic even if your finances do not permit you to purchase a wide variety of organic foods.The Dirty Dozen list identifies the twelve fruits and vegetables that, on average, contain the highest levels of contaminants. The following types of produce should be purchased organically first and foremost by you. The following 12 items make up the Dirty Dozen:

- Strawberries

- Spinach

- Nectarines

- Apples

- Grapes

- Peaches

- Cherries

- Pears

- Tomatoes

- Celery

- Potatoes

- Sweet bell peppers

The Environmental Working Group not only provides a list of the produce that tends to contain the most number of pesticides and pollutants, but they also provide a list of the produce that tendsto contain the lowest amount. You don't need to put as much of an emphasis on purchasing organic versions of these particular fruits and veggies. This list is known as the "Clean Fifteen," and the following items can be found on it:

- Avocados

- Corn on the cob

- Pineapples

- Cabbage

- Onions

- Frozen sweet peas

- Papayas

- Asparagus

- Mangos

- Eggplant

- Cantaloupe melon, honeydew

- Kiwis

- Cantaloupes

- Cauliflower

- Broccoli

7.10 Various Oils and Fats

There is no reason to be afraid of fat. In point of fact, having nutritious fats in your diet can supplyyou with useful vitamins and minerals and help you feel fuller for a longer period of time. The important thing is to pick fats that are healthy for you. Natural fats that are good for you are an essential part of any diet that is well-balanced.

Hydrogenated oils are the source of the trans fats that are found in margarine. Trans fats were developed to extend the shelf life of foods; nevertheless, research has shown that consumption of these fats can have a negative impact on cholesterol levels. Trans fats, on the other hand, raisethe levels of small, dense LDL particles, which are more likely to become lodged on the arterial walls and increase the risk of blockages that can lead to heart disease. Saturated fats, on the other hand, raise the levels of large, fluffy LDL particles that do not adhere to the arterial walls.

According to the Food and Drug Administration (FDA), there is a list of food ingredients that are "generally recognized as safe" (GRAS) and can be consumed by humans without risk. In 2015, the FDA took trans fats off of the list of substances that needed to be regulated and required foodmanufacturers to begin eliminating from their products any ingredients that included trans fats.

Omega-6 fatty acids are found in high concentrations in refined oils such as soybean oil, which isa component included in a wide variety of prepackaged foods. You are well aware that consuming an excessive amount of omega-6 fatty acids can contribute to chronic inflammation, which is linked to a number of diseases and other concerns relating to one's health.

These are some of the healthiest fats you can consume:

- Olive oil

- Avocado oil

- Unsalted grass-fed butter

- Ghee from grass-fed cows

- Coconut oil

- Walnut oil

- Hemp oil

- Sesame oil

Utilizing Fats in Cooking

There is a smoke point associated with every type of fat (a point at which they start to smoke when exposed to a certain temperature). The process of bringing lipids to their smoke point mightresult in the destruction of some of the fat's antioxidants and vitamins, as well as the production of substances that are detrimental to one's health. Particularly when cooking over a high heat, you need to be very careful to only use cooking oils that have a high smoke point in order to avoidburning the food. The oils and fats with the greatest smoke points, such as avocado oil, butter, ghee, and coconut oil, are the ones that work best in the kitchen. Olive oil can be used in cooking; however, it must be heated over a very low flame. It is recommended that walnut oil, hemp oil, andsesame oil be used for dressings or consumed when they are cool.

Additionally, keep fats in a cool, dark place away from any sources of heat. The heat that is left over from cooking can cause lipids to develop rancid if they are kept in close proximity to a stove or oven.

7.10.2 Sugar and Sweeteners

Sugar, not fat, is the primary cause of the majority of the health problems that people are quick toblame on fat. Despite the absence of any beneficial effects on human health, the typical annual sugar intake for an American is roughly 66 pounds. Even more worrisome than the fact that sugarhas no nutritional value is the fact that it adds to chronic inflammation, raises your risk of heart disease, destabilizes blood sugar levels, and feeds cancer cells. These are all conditions that are associated with poor health. Consuming an excessive amount of sugar may also make it simplerfor you to put on weight.

Studies have shown that people who consume artificial sweeteners have a higher risk of developing diabetes, metabolic syndrome, and cardiovascular disease. Despite the fact that manufacturers have tried to solve the problem of sugar by introducing artificial sweeteners to the market, the problem still remains. Additionally, artificial sweeteners can upset the natural balance of microorganisms in your gut, which can lead to gastrointestinal and even systemic problems.

Additionally, artificial sweeteners have been associated with an increased risk of developing cancer as well as chronic migraines. In addition to this, giving your body the sensation of sweetness without providing it with any calories might result in cravings for sugar that are even stronger than they were before.

Sugar, in any of its many forms, should have as little of an impact on one's diet as is humanly possible. However, some sweeteners are healthier for you to consume than others are, and this is not always the case. The following are some of the better options:

• Pure maple syrup

• Raw honey

• Coconut sugar

• Date sugar

• Monk fruit

• Molasses

• Stevia

• Erythritol

7.10.3 A Remark Concerning Stevia

Even though stevia comes from plants and is sold as a natural sweetener, many of the packagedforms have undergone extensive processing before being made available to consumers like you.In addition to this, several stevia products include other, undesirable components, such as "natural flavors," among their list of constituents. Companies are permitted to use the label "natural flavors" even when their products contain chemical additions that simulate natural flavorssince the FDA does not strictly regulate the use of the term "natural flavors." If you do decide to use stevia, make sure you only use a very small amount of it and pick a brand that is 100 percentnatural and organic.

Chapter 8

The Do's and Don'ts

While intermittent fasting can have many potential benefits, it is important to approach it with caution and understanding of both the do's and don'ts. In this chapter, I will discuss the various types of intermittent fasting, the potential benefits and drawbacks, and provide guidelines for safely incorporating intermittent fasting into your lifestyle.

It's important to note that intermittent fasting is not a one-size-fits-all solution, and what may workfor one person may not work for another. It's crucial to consult with a healthcare professional before starting any new eating pattern, especially if you have any underlying health conditions or take medications that may be affected by changes in your diet. Each type of intermittent fasting has its own set of do's and don'ts to consider.

8.1 Ease into the fast gradually

Start out slowly so that your body has time to adjust to the new food routine. Altering one's diet or way of life drastically can generate a variety of unpleasant side effects, some of which may discourage one from pursuing a healthier lifestyle.

This is especially true for more advanced forms of intermittent fasting, such as the One Meal a Day plan, as well as for longer periods of time spent fasting. For some people, even a gradual transition to intermittent fasting 16/8 with a 16-hour fasting period followed by an 8-hour eating window might trigger headaches, weariness, dizziness, and make it difficult to maintain control over their hunger levels.

In light of this, I recommend beginning the practice gradually. You would begin with a 12/12 schedule and gradually increase the amount of time spent fasting by one hour per day until you finally reached a 16/8 schedule. This strategy lessens the severity of the negative effects and teaches you more about how your body responds to the intermittent fasting regimen.

8.2 Your routine of intermittent fasting should not be altered

When it comes to intermittent fasting, consistency is essential. Maintaining a consistent fasting window throughout the day will make it easier for you to implement intermittent fasting into your lifestyle. It will become ingrained in your routine and become a habit, which will increase the likelihood that you will continue doing it and be successful.

Naturally, the ordinary lives we lead might be unpredictable at times, and we must be flexible withour plans. Try not to give in to discouragement and start again the following day. In circumstances like these, it is of the utmost importance to have a routine that has already been established andthat functions well for you.

8.3 Make sure to stay hydrated.

Because water makes up to 60 percent of the human body, maintaining proper hydration is always extremely important.

There are a lot of reasons why you should drink water, but one of the most important ones is thatit can become your closest buddy during fasting hours. It will not only make the skin look better, purge the body of toxins, and make you feel more invigorated, but it will also decrease your appetite. There is some evidence that drinking water can reduce the feeling of hunger, and one glass of water can be an effective approach to do so.

8.4 During a fast, you shouldn't consume any drinks with zerocalories or artificial sweeteners.

When you fast, you don't consume any food or drinks that contain calories. Does this imply that consuming a diet soda will not add any calories to your diet? This is a question that frequently arises among those who are just starting out with intermittent fasting. During a fast, it is generallyrecommended to abstain from using artificial sweeteners and to avoid drinking diet sodas.

According to a number of studies, using artificial sweeteners can make you feel hungry, which inturn may cause you to consume more food. Within the realm of artificial sweeteners and their effects on the body, insulin response, blood sugar levels, and the influence they have on gut bacteria, there is a great deal of knowledge and research that is contradictory to one another.

As a result, it is recommended to limit one's beverage consumption to beverages that have beenshown to be compatible with intermittent fasting, such as water, unsweetened tea, and black coffee. To view the definitive list of drinks suitable for intermittent fasting, go here.

8.5 Review your diet while you are conducting intermittent fasting

Technically speaking, intermittent fasting does not include limiting the kind of foods that you consume but rather the times during which you consume food. However, if you want to reduce weight, you need also examine the foods that you eat and how much you are eating of them.

A good rule of thumb for maintaining a healthy diet is to eat a greater variety of whole foods, reduce the amount of sugar and saturated fat you consume, and make sure that the majority of your meals consist of vegetables and fruits.

You can also give one of these meal plans for intermittent fasting for 21 days a shot to see if it helps you maintain a healthy and well-balanced diet. You can select from a wide variety of calorie possibilities, as well as six distinct types of diets: standard, keto, vegan keto, vegetarian, vegan, and paleo diets.

8.6 In order to maintain your weight loss while engaging inintermittent fasting, you can't consume anything you want

It is still feasible to ingest the same number of calories in the same length of time, despite the factthat it is technically more difficult to do so. You could be consuming a lot of calories, which will not help you lose weight. This is especially true if your diet is high in saturated fat, which can come from oils, red meat, and fast food. You could also be consuming a lot of empty calories, which can come from sugary drinks, sweets, and alcohol. In addition, these won't be foods that are very high in nutritive value, in the sense that they include a lot of vitamins, minerals, fiber, orantioxidants.

A balanced diet is therefore required in order to achieve sustainable weight loss that is also beneficial to the health of the body.

8.7 Prepare yourself for the hunger sensation

Intermittent fasting often results in feelings of hunger. The good news is that with enough practice,you'll eventually figure out how to manage the hunger that comes with fasting and limit its effects.

From consuming large amounts of water or a cup of coffee black, to learning how to avoid food cravings, to scheduling busy meetings or workouts during the fasting window, there are a variety of strategies that can be utilized. There are a variety of strategies that can be utilized to get through some challenging fasting hours. You just need to figure out what works best for you andstick with that.

8.8 Don't put undue strain on yourself

There are instances when practicing intermittent fasting can be difficult. However, you should train yourself to pay attention to your body so that you can determine when you need to rest. When you are fasting, you should exercise with an extra level of caution. Maintain a lower intensity for your workouts while you are in the fasting window, and schedule your cardio or strength training for when you are in the eating window.

It may be more difficult to maintain the fast during specific phases of a woman's menstrual cycle for women who practice intermittent fasting. In addition, certain women are more susceptible to shifts in their diet and lifestyle, which can throw off their hormones and interrupt their cycle.

In situations like these, or if you are feeling fatigued, dizzy, or have a headache and taking rest or staying hydrated does not help, you should think about reducing the amount of time you spend fasting or reviewing your diet to ensure that you are getting enough protein and healthy fats in your meals.

8.9 Have fun with the process of your intermittent fasting

Although losing weight is a fantastic benefit of intermittent fasting, another major benefit is the feeling of empowerment that comes from taking control of your urges. Many individuals also report feeling more focused, having more energy, having better sleep, and generally just reporting that they feel and look better overall. Even after only a few weeks of practicing intermittent fasting, one can see these changes taking place in their bodies.

The practice of intermittent fasting can become an essential component of one's daily routine, and considering this fact should not be something that causes mental anguish. As a result, it is essential to choose the type of intermittent fasting schedule that is most suitable for you, as well as to discover a way to limit the adverse effects, lessen feelings of hunger, and maintain a diet that is both healthy and balanced so that your body is well nourished.

8.10 Don't forget to seek answers to your queries and make yourlifestyle of intermittent fasting better

If you are already here reading about the dos and don'ts of intermittent fasting, then you are already ahead of the game. It is essential to maintain an inquisitive mindset and strive for continuous improvement. There is a wealth of information available on intermittent fasting, rangingfrom books on the topic to blogs written by specialists on the subject who share their insights and personal experiences with fasting.

Chapter 9

30 days training program

Now that you have a better understanding of what intermittent fasting is and how it can benefit women, it's time to start your 30-day training program. Here are some tips to help you get started:

- Choose a fasting schedule that works for you: As mentioned earlier, the most popular method of intermittent fasting is the 16/8 method, which involves fasting for 16 hours and eating during an 8-hour window. However, this may not work for everyone. If you are new to intermittent fasting, you may want to start with a shorter fasting period, such as 14 hours, and gradually work your way up to 16 hours. It's important to find a schedule that works for you and that you can stick with.

- Drink plenty of water: It's important to stay hydrated while intermittent fasting, especially during the fasting periods. Aim to drink at least 8 cups of water per day, and more if you are exercising or sweating heavily.

- Eat nourishing foods during your eating window: Intermittent fasting is not a license to eat unhealthy foods during your eating window. It's important to focus on nourishing, whole foods that provide your body with the nutrients it needs. This includes plenty of fruits and vegetables, lean proteins, and healthy fats. Avoid processed, sugary, and high-fat foods as much as possible.

- Don't overeat during your eating window: It can be tempting to overindulge during your eating window, especially if you are feeling hungry after a long fast. However, it's important to remember that the goal of intermittent fasting is not to eat as much as possible during your eating window, but rather to limit your overall calorie intake. Be mindful of portion sizes and try to eat slowly and mindfully.

- Be consistent: Intermittent fasting works best when you are consistent with your fasting schedule. Try to stick to the same eating and fasting times every day to make it a habit.

Now that you have a basic understanding of how to get started with intermittent fasting, it's time to dive into the 30-day plan. This plan is designed to gradually introduce you to the concept of intermittent fasting and help you build the habit over the course of a month.

9.1 The schedule

9.1.1 Week One: 16/8 Method

<u>Week 1</u>

GOAL

Our goal for this week is to successfully implement the 16/8 method of intermittent fasting intoour daily routine. To achieve this goal, here are a few tips to keep in mind:

• Choose a consistent window of time for your fasting and feeding periods. Many peoplefind it helpful to fast for 16 hours and eat during an 8-hour window, such as from noon to 8pm.

• Drink plenty of water during your fasting period to help curb hunger and keep your bodyhydrated.

• Incorporate low-calorie, nutrient-dense foods into your meals to help you feel satisfied and nourished during the eating window.

• Be mindful of portion sizes and choose healthy, whole foods to support your overall health and wellness goals.

• Allow yourself some flexibility and grace as you adjust to this new way of eating. It may take a little time to get used to, but with practice and patience, you can successfully incorporate the 16/8 method into your lifestyle.

Monday

- 11 a.m.: Autumn Breakfast Chia Bowl (a bowl of chia seeds mixed with autumn-inspired ingredients such as pumpkin puree, diced apples, and cinnamon)

- 1 p.m.: Stuffed Eggs (hard-boiled eggs filled with a mixture of cheese, vegetables, and protein of choice)

- 3 p.m.: Spicy Shrimp with Lemon Yogurt on Wilted Greens (shrimp cooked with spices served on a bed of wilted greens with a lemon yogurt sauce)

- 5 p.m.: Spinach and Feta-Stuffed Chicken Breasts (chicken breasts stuffed with a mixture of spinach and feta cheese)

- 6:30 p.m.: Sugar-Free No-Bake Cocoa Balls (balls made with cocoa powder, nuts, and sweeteners of choice, rolled in coconut or nuts)

Tuesday

- 11 a.m.: Flourless Cinnamon Banana Pancakes (pancakes made with mashed bananas and cinnamon, without flour)

- 1 p.m.: Salsa Fresca with Plantain Chips (fresh salsa made with diced tomatoes, onions, and peppers served with fried or baked plantain chips)

- 3 p.m.: Traditional Greek Salad (a salad with lettuce, tomatoes, cucumbers, olives, andfeta cheese, dressed with olive oil and lemon juice)

- 5 p.m.: Lemon Thyme Chicken (chicken breasts cooked with lemon and thyme)

- 6:30 p.m.: Easy Banana Date Cookies (cookies made with mashed bananas, dates, andoats)

Wednesday

- 11 a.m.: Chicken Sausage Patties and Vegetarian Hash (chicken sausage patties served with a hash made with vegetables of choice)

- 1 p.m.: Cinnamon Spice Granola (homemade granola made with oats, nuts, seeds, andspices)

- 3 p.m.: Dandelion and White Bean Soup (a soup made with dandelion greens and whitebeans)

- 5 p.m.: Pork and Fennel Meatballs (meatballs made with ground pork and fennel seeds)

- 6:30 p.m.: Strawberry Coconut Ice Cream (ice cream made with coconut milk and freshstrawberries)

Thursday

- 11 a.m.: Overnight Almond Butter Pumpkin Spice Oats (overnight oats made with almondbutter, pumpkin puree, and pumpkin spice)

- 1 p.m.: Mini Baked Eggplant Pizza Bites (bite-sized eggplant slices topped with tomato sauce, cheese, and toppings of choice, baked in the oven)

- 3 p.m.: Wild Rice Salad with Mushrooms and Almonds (a salad made with wild rice, mushrooms, almonds, and a dressing of choice)

- 5 p.m.: Stuffed Peppers with Ground Turkey (bell peppers stuffed with a mixture of ground turkey and vegetables)

- 6:30 p.m.: Chocolate Coconut-Milk Cubes (frozen cubes made with coconut milk and cocoa powder)

Friday

- 11 a.m.: Huevos Rancheros Without Tortillas (eggs cooked in a spicy tomato sauce, served without tortillas)

- 1 p.m.: Cranberry Almond Granola (homemade granola made with oats, nuts, seeds, and cranberries)

- 3 p.m.: Lentil Salad (a salad made with lentils, vegetables, and a dressing of choice)

- 5 p.m.: Citrus Flank Steak (flank steak marinated in a citrus juice and served with vegetables)

- 6:30 p.m.: Almond Butter Cookies (cookies made with almond butter, oats, and sweeteners of choice)

Saturday

- 11 a.m.: Gut-Friendly Smoothie (a smoothie made with

ingredients that support gut health,such as probiotics, fiber, and fermented foods)

- 1 p.m.: Garlicky Parsnip and Carrot Fries (parsnip and carrot slices baked in the oven withgarlic and herbs)

- 3 p.m.: Butter Lettuce Salad with Poached Eggs and Bacon (a salad made with butterlettuce and topped with poached eggs and bacon)

- 5 p.m.: Chicken Burgers (burgers made with ground chicken and seasonings of choice)

- 6:30 p.m.: Heavenly Cookie Bars (bars made with oats, nuts, and dried fruit)

Sunday

- 11 a.m.: Farmers' Scrambler (scrambled eggs with a variety of vegetables and protein ofchoice)

- 1 p.m.: Chocolate Chip Energy Bites (energy balls made with oats, nuts, and chocolatechips)

- 3 p.m.: Tarragon Lemon Chicken (chicken breasts cooked with tarragon and lemon)

- 5 p.m.: Fish Curry (a curry made with fish and vegetables, flavored with Indian spices)

- 6:30 p.m.: Delicious Pumpkin Pudding (pudding made with pumpkin puree and spices)

SELF-REFLECTION

What I did great 👍	What I need to work on 👎
_____	_____
_____	_____
_____	_____
_____	_____
_____	_____
_____	_____
_____	_____
_____	_____
_____	_____

★ OVERALL SCORE (1-5) ★

9.1.2 Week Two: Eat-Stop-Eat Method

Week 2

GOAL

For week two of intermittent fasting training using the eat-stop-eat method, your goal is to continue building your fasting endurance and increasing the duration of your fasts. Here are some tips to help you succeed:

• Gradually increase the length of your fasts: Start by adding an extra day of fasting to your schedule each week. For example, if you were fasting for 24 hours on Monday andThursday in week one, aim to fast for 24 hours on Monday, Thursday, and Saturday inweek two.

• Stay hydrated: Drink plenty of water, herbal tea, and other non-caloric beverages duringyour eating periods to help you stay hydrated and avoid dehydration during your fasts.

• Don't skip meals: It's important to eat well during your eating periods to ensure you're getting all the nutrients your body needs. Don't skip meals or skimp on portion sizes, asthis can negatively impact your energy levels and overall health.

• Get plenty of rest: Fasting can be physically and mentally demanding, so be sure to getplenty of rest and sleep to help you recover and stay energized.

• Stay motivated: Intermittent fasting can be challenging, so it's important to stay motivated and focused on your goals. Consider enlisting the support of a friend or familymember to help you stay on track or keep a food and exercise journal to track your progress.

Monday

• Breakfast: Very Vegetable Frittata (a frittata made with a variety of vegetables)

• Snack: Beet the Bloat (a smoothie made with beets and other ingredients to supportdigestion)

• Lunch: Turkey Meatballs (meatballs made with ground turkey and seasonings of choice)

• Dinner: Slow Cooker Chicken Tagine (a Moroccan dish made with chicken, vegetables,and spices, cooked in a slow cooker)

• Dessert: Paleo Chocolate Bars (chocolate bars made with cocoa powder and sweetenersthat are compliant with the paleo diet)

Tuesday

• Breakfast: Pumpkin Spice Smoothie (a smoothie made with pumpkin puree and spices)

• Snack: Broccoli, Pine Nut, and Apple Salad (a salad made with broccoli, pine nuts, andapples, dressed with a vinaigrette)

• Lunch: Coconut-Crumbed Chicken (chicken coated in coconut and fried or baked)

• Dinner: Tuscan White Bean Soup (a soup made with white beans, tomatoes, and herbs)

• Dessert: Banana Coconut "Nice" Cream (frozen banana blended with coconut milk to create a creamy, ice cream-like consistency)

Wednesday

FAST (no eating for 24 hours)

Thursday

• Breakfast: Strawberry Banana Pancake (pancakes made with mashed bananas andstrawberries)

• Snack: Stuffed Mushroom Caps (mushroom caps stuffed with a filling of choice)

• Lunch: Chicken Soup with Asparagus (a soup made with chicken and asparagus)

• Dinner: Eggplant Parmigiana (eggplant slices breaded and baked with tomato sauce andcheese)

• Dessert: Paleo Fudge (fudge made with paleo-approved ingredients such as nuts andcocoa powder)

Friday

FAST (no eating for 24 hours)

Saturday

• Breakfast: Raspberry Banana Mint Chia Pudding (chia seeds soaked in milk and mixedwith raspberries, banana, and mint)

• Snack: Avocado Salad (a salad made with avocado and other vegetables, dressed with avinaigrette)

• Lunch: Chickpeas in Potato Onion Curry (a curry made with chickpeas, potatoes, onions,and Indian spices)

• Dinner: Marinated London Broil (London broil marinated in a mixture of oil, vinegar, andspices)

• Dessert: Peanut Butter Cookies (cookies made with peanut butter and sweeteners ofchoice)

Sunday

• Breakfast: Pineapple Turmeric Smoothie (a smoothie made with pineapple and turmeric)

• Snack: Blueberry Chia Seed Jam with Gluten-Free Crackers (homemade jam made withblueberries and chia seeds served with gluten-free crackers)

• Lunch: California Garden Salad with Avocado and Sprouts (a salad made with avocado,sprouts, and a variety of vegetables)

• Dinner: Lamb Patties (patties made with ground lamb and seasonings of choice)

• Dessert: Raspberry Lemon Oatmeal Bars (bars made with oats, raspberries, lemon, andsweeteners of choice)

SELF-REFLECTION

What I did great 👍	What I need to work on 👎
_____	_____
_____	_____
_____	_____
_____	_____
_____	_____
_____	_____
_____	_____
_____	_____
_____	_____

★ OVERALL SCORE (1-5) ★

9.1.3 Week Three: 5:2 Method

Week 3

GOAL

The goal of week three of intermittent fasting training using the 5:2 method is to continue to develop a consistent eating pattern that allows for periods of fasting and feasting. Here are some tips to help you succeed:

- Plan ahead: Make sure you have healthy, low-calorie options available for your fasting days, and make sure you have enough food for your feasting days.

- Stay hydrated: Drink plenty of water and other calorie-free beverages during your fastingperiods to help curb hunger and keep your energy levels up.

- Eat mindfully: On your feasting days, pay attention to your food and try to eat slowly tohelp you feel full and satisfied.

- Exercise regularly: Incorporating regular physical activity into your routine can help youfeel energized and improve your overall health.

- Monitor your progress: Keep track of your weight and other markers of progress, such as measurements or how you feel, to help you stay motivated and make any necessary adjustments to your plan.

The goal of week three of intermittent fasting training using the 5:2 method is to continue to develop a consistent eating pattern that allows for periods of fasting and feasting. Here are some tips to help you succeed:

- Plan ahead: Make sure you have healthy, low-calorie options available for your fasting days, and make sure you have enough food for your feasting days.

- Stay hydrated: Drink plenty of water and other calorie-free beverages during your fastingperiods to help curb hunger and keep your energy levels up.

- Eat mindfully: On your feasting days, pay attention to your food and try to eat slowly tohelp you feel full and satisfied.

- Exercise regularly: Incorporating regular physical activity into your routine can help youfeel energized and improve your overall health.

- Monitor your progress: Keep track of your weight and other markers of progress, such as measurements or how you feel, to help you stay motivated and make any necessary adjustments to your plan.

Monday

- Breakfast: Pumpkin Spice Smoothie (a smoothie made with pumpkin puree and spices)

- Snack: Sardines in Red Pepper Cups (sardines served in red pepper cups, seasoned withherbs and spices)

- Lunch: Turkey Meatballs with Roasted Beet Slaw (meatballs made with ground turkey andserved with a slaw made with roasted beets)

- Dinner: Mediterranean Flaky Fish with Vegetables (a fish dish cooked with Mediterraneanspices and served with vegetables)

- Dessert: Peppermint Patties (homemade peppermint patties made with paleo-approvedingredients)

Tuesday

- Breakfast: Roasted Vegetable Frittata (a frittata made with roasted vegetables)

- Snack: Broccoli, Pine Nut, and Apple Salad (a salad made with broccoli, pine nuts, andapples, dressed with a vinaigrette)

- Lunch: Chicken Soup with Asparagus (a soup made with chicken and asparagus)

- Dinner: Lentil-Stuffed Peppers (peppers stuffed with a mixture of lentils and otheringredients)

- Dessert: Blueberry Pie (pie made with fresh or frozen blueberries and a paleo-approvedcrust)

Fasting Day

- Meal One: Curried Shrimp with Vegetables (shrimp cooked with curry spices and servedwith vegetables)

- Meal Two: Pepper Steak (steak cooked with peppers and other vegetables)

Thursday

- Breakfast: Salmon Omelet (an omelet made with salmon and vegetables)

- Snack: Paleo Chips with Onion Jam (homemade chips made with paleo-approvedingredients served with onion jam)

- Lunch: South American Chili (a chili made with South American spices and a variety ofbeans and vegetables)

- Dinner: Beef with Spinach and Sweet Potatoes (beef served with sautéed spinach andsweet potatoes)

- Dessert: Maple Rice Pudding with Walnuts (rice pudding made with maple syrup andserved with walnuts)

Fasting Day

- Meal One: Pumpkin Maple Roast Chicken (chicken roasted with pumpkin puree and maplesyrup)

- Meal Two: Lentil-Stuffed Peppers (peppers stuffed with a mixture of lentils and otheringredients)

Saturday

- Breakfast: Bacon and Vegetable Omelet (an omelet made with bacon and vegetables)

• Snack: Chocolate Chip Energy Bites (homemade energy bites made with chocolate chipsand other ingredients)

• Lunch: Tarragon Lemon Chicken (chicken cooked with tarragon and lemon)

• Dinner: Zoodles with Pesto (zucchini noodles served with pesto sauce)

• Dessert: Banana Sorbet (sorbet made with frozen bananas and other ingredients)

Sunday

• Breakfast: Autumn Breakfast Chia Bowl (a bowl made with chia seeds, autumnal fruitsand spices)

• Snack: Chocolate Chip Energy Bites (homemade energy bites made with chocolate chipsand other ingredients)

• Lunch: Picadillo (a Cuban dish made with ground beef and vegetables)

• Dinner: Fish Curry (a curry made with fish and Indian spices)

• Dessert: Baked Apples (apples baked with a filling of choice)

Melissa May

SELF-REFLECTION

What I did great 👍	What I need to work on 👎
_____	_____
_____	_____
_____	_____
_____	_____
_____	_____
_____	_____
_____	_____
_____	_____
_____	_____

★ OVERALL SCORE (1-5) ★

9.1.4 Week Four +2 days: Alternate Day Method

Week 4

GOAL

For the final week of intermittent fasting training using the alternate day method, our goal is to continue following the protocol consistently, making sure to plan our meals and snacks in advance to ensure we are properly nourished. It's important to listen to our bodies and make adjustments as needed, such as taking an extra day off if we are feeling particularly hungry or fatigued. Here are a few tips to help you succeed during this final week

• Plan ahead: As mentioned, it's important to plan our meals and snacks in advance to make sure we are properly nourished during our eating periods. This can help prevent overindulging and make it easier to stick to our fast days.

• Stay hydrated: Make sure to drink plenty of water during your eating periods to help keep hunger at bay and support overall hydration.

• Exercise regularly: Exercise can help boost metabolism and increase feelings offullness, making it a helpful tool for sticking to our intermittent fasting plan. Just be sureto listen to your body and adjust your workout intensity as needed.

• Seek support: If you're finding it difficult to stick to the plan, consider seeking support from friends, family, or a healthcare professional. Sometimes having a supportive network can make all the difference in helping us achieve our goals.

- Keep track of progress: It can be helpful to keep track of our progress during this final week of intermittent fasting training. This could involve taking measurements, keeping a food diary, or tracking how we feel during our fast days. This can help us see the progress we have made and identify any areas where we may need to make adjustments. It can also be helpful to reflect on any challenges or successes we have experienced during the training process and consider how we can apply these lessonsmoving forward.

Fasting Day

- Meal One: Artichoke and Cheese Squares (squares made with artichoke and cheese)

- Meal Two: Slow Cooker Chicken Tagine (a Moroccan dish made with chicken, vegetables,and spices, cooked in a slow cooker)

Tuesday

- Breakfast: Roasted Vegetable Frittata (a frittata made with roasted vegetables)

- Snack: Mini Baked Eggplant Pizza Bites (mini pizzas made with eggplant slices as thecrust)

- Lunch: Coconut-Crumbed Chicken (chicken coated in coconut and fried or baked)

- Dinner: Zucchini "Lasagna" (lasagna made with zucchini slices instead of pasta)

- Dessert: Almond Butter Cookies (cookies made with almond butter and sweeteners ofchoice)

Fasting Day

• Meal One: Tomato and Leek Frittata (a frittata made with tomato and leek)

• Meal Two: Paleo Stuffed Peppers (peppers stuffed with a paleo-approved filling)

Thursday

• Breakfast: Gut-Friendly Smoothie (a smoothie made with ingredients to support digestion)

• Snack: Beet the Bloat (a smoothie made with beets and other ingredients to supportdigestion)

• Lunch: Pumpkin Soup with Caraway Seeds (a soup made with pumpkin and carawayseeds)

• Dinner: Filet Mignon Salad (a salad made with filet mignon and vegetables)

• Dessert: Apricot Ginger Sorbet (sorbet made with apricots and ginger)

Fasting Day

• Meal One: Bacon and Vegetable Omelet (an omelet made with bacon and vegetables)

• Meal Two: Picadillo (a Cuban dish made with ground beef and vegetables)

Saturday

• Breakfast: Strawberry Banana Pancake (pancakes made with mashed bananas andstrawberries)

• Snack: Avocado Salad (a salad made with avocado and other vegetables, dressed with avinaigrette)

• Lunch: Chickpeas in Potato Onion Curry (a curry made with chickpeas, potatoes, onions,and Indian spices)

• Dinner: Easy Pan Chicken (chicken made with a simple marinade and cooked in a pan)

• Dessert: Fruit Salad with Ginger and Lemon Juice (a fruit salad made with a variety offruits and seasoned with ginger and lemon juice)

Fasting Day

• Meal One: Garlicky Vegetable-Packed Omelet (an omelet made with vegetables andseasoned with garlic)

• Meal Two: Lamb Patties (patties made with ground lamb and seasoned with herbs andspices)

Monday

• Breakfast: Roasted Vegetable Frittata (a frittata made with roasted vegetables)

• Snack: Mini Baked Eggplant Pizza Bites (mini pizzas made with eggplant slices as thecrust)

• Lunch: Coconut-Crumbed Chicken (chicken coated in coconut and fried or baked)

• Dinner: Zucchini "Lasagna" (lasagna made with zucchini slices instead of pasta)

• Dessert: Almond Butter Cookies (cookies made with almond butter and sweeteners ofchoice)

Fasting Day

• Meal One: Tomato and Leek Frittata (a frittata made with tomato and leek)

• Meal Two: Paleo Stuffed Peppers (peppers stuffed with a paleo-approved filling)

SELF-REFLECTION

What I did great 👍	What I need to work on 👎
_____	_____
_____	_____
_____	_____
_____	_____
_____	_____
_____	_____
_____	_____
_____	_____
_____	_____

★ OVERALL SCORE (1-5) ★

9.2 Eating and calories

9.2.1 How much should you eat?

When it comes to determining how much to eat after a period of fasting, it is important to listen to your body's hunger and fullness cues. It is generally recommended to eat until you feel satisfied, but not overly full or stuffed. This is because overeating can lead to weight gain and other negative health consequences. It is also important to choose nutrient-dense, whole foods as part of your meals and to pay attention to portion sizes. This will help ensure that you are meeting your nutritional needs and supporting your overall health and well-being.

To help you keep track of your food intake and make sure you are meeting your nutritional needs, it may be helpful to use a food diary or a tracking app. These tools can help you keep track of the types and amounts of foods you are eating, as well as the number of calories you are consuming. It is important to remember that everyone is different, and it is important to find an eating pattern that works best for you and your individual needs and goals.

10.2.2 What should you be mindful of when eating?

When it comes to eating, there are several things that you should be mindful of in order to support your health and well-being. Here are some key points to consider:

1. **Chew slowly:** Taking the time to chew your food thoroughly can help you feel more satisfied and may even help you eat less. It can also help improve your digestion andnutrient absorption.

2. **Pay attention to your hunger and fullness cues:** Paying attention to your body'shunger and fullness cues can help you tune into your body's needs and prevent overeating. Try to stop eating when you feel satisfied, rather than stuffed.

3. **Choose nutrient-dense, whole foods:** Focusing on whole, nutrient-dense foods can help you get the nutrients your body needs to function properly and support your overallhealth. This means choosing foods that are high in vitamins, minerals, and fiber and lowin added sugars, sodium, and unhealthy fats.

4. **Portion sizes:** Paying attention to portion sizes can help you maintain a healthy weightand prevent overeating. It can be helpful to use measuring cups or a food scale to helpyou measure out appropriate portion sizes.

5. **Hydration:** Staying hydrated is important for overall health and well-being. Aim to drinkplenty of water throughout the day and try to limit sugary beverages.

6. **Mindful eating:** Practicing mindful eating can help you pay more attention to your foodand the eating experience. This can involve things like eating without distractions, savoring your food, and paying attention to your thoughts and emotions while eating.

By being mindful of these points while eating, you can support your health and well-being anddevelop a healthy relationship with food.

9.2.3 What is a calorie?

A calorie is a unit of energy that is used to measure the energy content of foods. When we talk about food and nutrition, calories refer to the energy that is stored in the food that we eat. The body uses calories from food to fuel all of its functions, including physical activity, digestion, andorgan function.

The number of calories that a person needs can vary depending on their age, sex, weight, height, and physical activity level. For example, a sedentary adult woman may need fewer calories than an active adult man. It is generally recommended that adults aim for a daily intakeof 2000-2500 calories per day, although this can vary depending on individual needs and goals.For example, people who are trying to lose weight may need to consume fewer calories, while those who are trying to gain weight or build muscle may need to consume more calories.

It is important to pay attention to the number of calories you are consuming and to choose nutrient-dense, whole foods to help meet your nutritional needs. This means choosing foods that are high in nutrients like vitamins, minerals, and fiber and low in added sugars, sodium, andunhealthy fats. By focusing on nutrient-dense foods, you can ensure that you are getting the nutrients your body needs to function properly while also helping to maintain a healthy weight.

9.2.4 Caloric requirements and maintenance

To gain weight, the general rule of thumb is to aim for an additional 250-500 calories per day. This can help a person gradually gain weight over time. It is important to choose nutrient-dense, whole foods as part of this calorie increase to ensure that the weight gain is healthy and sustainable.

To lose weight, the general rule of thumb is to aim for a deficit of 500-1000 calories per day. This can help a person gradually lose weight over time. It is important to choose nutrient-dense,whole foods as part of this calorie reduction to ensure that the weight loss is healthy and sustainable.

It is important to note that weight loss and weight gain are not always simple and can be influenced by many factors beyond just calorie intake. For example, genetics, hormone imbalances, and other medical conditions can all affect a person's weight. It is always a good idea to speak with a healthcare professional before making any significant changes to your dietor exercise routine.

9.2.5 Weight loss examples

Example 1:

If you weigh 200 pounds and want to shed 10 pounds in 5 weeks, a safe and sustainable rate of weight loss is 1 pound per week. To achieve this, you'll need to create a calorie deficit of around 500 calories per day. This can be done through a combination of diet and exercise.

If you aim for a daily calorie intake of 1500, this would create a deficit of 500 calories (2500 maintenance calories - 1500 calorie intake = 1000 calorie deficit/week). This deficit would help you lose 1 pound per week, allowing you to reach your target weight loss of 10 pounds in 5 weeks.

Example 2:

If you weigh 150 pounds and are hoping to lose 5 pounds in 2 weeks, a healthy rate of weight loss is 0.5 pounds per week. To achieve this, you'll need to create a calorie deficit of approximately 250 calories per day.

For example, if you aim for a daily calorie intake of 1250, this will create a deficit of 250 calories (1750 maintenance calories - 1250 calorie intake = 500 calorie deficit/week). This deficit would help you lose 0.5 pounds per week, allowing you to reach your target weight loss of 5 pounds in 2 weeks.

Example 3:

If you weigh 180 pounds and are looking to shed 15 pounds over the course of 8 weeks, a healthy rate of weight loss is 1.875 pounds per week. To achieve this, you'll need to create acalorie deficit of about 938 calories per day.

For instance, if you aim for a daily calorie intake of 1062, this will create a deficit of 938 calories (2000 maintenance calories - 1062 calorie intake = 938 calorie deficit/week). This deficitwould help you lose 1.875 pounds per week, allowing you to reach your target weight loss of 15 pounds in 8 weeks.

Weight Loss Quiz

If you're a woman interested in trying intermittent fasting to achieve your weight loss goals, it's important to find the right number of calories for you to eat in order to see success. The good news is that you can easily determine the exact number of calories you need to eat based on your metabolism, activity level, and time frame using our quiz at the link provided. Simply follow the prompts and you'll have all the details you need to get started on your weight loss journey with intermittent fasting.

Scan Here:

SCAN ME

9.3 Tips for success

As you work your way through the 30-day intermittent fasting program, here are a few tips to helpyou stay on track and achieve success:

• Plan your meals: It can be helpful to plan out your meals in advance to make sure you aregetting enough nourishment during your eating window. This can also help you avoid thetemptation to reach for unhealthy foods when you are feeling hungry.

• Don't skip meals: It's important to eat during your eating window, even if you are not feelingparticularly hungry. Skipping meals can make it harder to stick to your fasting schedule and may cause you to feel weak or sluggish.

• Listen to your body: Intermittent fasting is not right for everyone, and it's important to listento your body and pay attention to how you are feeling. If you are feeling excessively hungryor tired, or if you are experiencing any other negative side effects, it may be necessary toadjust your fasting schedule or consider a different approach to weight loss and health.

• Stay active: Exercise can be a great way to boost weight loss and improve overall healthwhile intermittent fasting. Try to incorporate some form of physical activity into your daily routine, whether it's a brisk walk, a yoga class, or a high-intensity interval training (HIIT)

workout. Just be sure to listen to your body and don't push yourself too hard, especially ifyou are new to exercise or have any underlying health conditions.

Don't get discouraged: Intermittent fasting can be challenging at times, and it's normal to have setbacks or moments of temptation. If you slip up or have a less-than-perfect day, don't get discouraged. Just get back on track and keep going. Remember, the key to success with intermittent fasting is consistency.

9.4 Troubleshooting Common Issues with Intermittent Fasting

While intermittent fasting can be an effective and beneficial eating pattern, it's not without its challenges. Here are some common issues that may arise and how to troubleshoot them:

• Hunger: It's normal to feel hungry during the fasting periods, especially at first. If you are struggling with hunger, try drinking plenty of water, eating filling and nourishing foods during your eating window, and engaging in physical activity to help reduce hunger pangs.You may also want to consider gradually increasing your fasting period over time to help your body adjust.

• Low energy: If you are feeling weak or sluggish while intermittent fasting, it may be due tolow blood sugar or insufficient calorie intake. Try eating more balanced meals during youreating window and incorporating more healthy fats and proteins to help keep your energylevels stable.

• Difficulty sticking to the plan: It can be tough to stick to any new eating pattern, and intermittent fasting is no exception. If you are having difficulty sticking to your fasting schedule, try to identify any triggers or obstacles that may be causing you to stray from the plan. It may also be helpful to enlist the support of a friend or family member to help you stay motivated and on track.

9.5 Conclusion

Congratulations on completing our 30-day intermittent fasting training program for women! We hope that this program has helped you understand the basics of intermittent fasting and providedyou with the tools and resources you need to make it a part of your long-term health and wellnessplan. Remember, the key to success with intermittent fasting is consistency and patience. It maytake some time for your body to adjust to the new eating pattern, but with dedication and perseverance, you can achieve your health and weight loss goals.

Chapter 10

Myths and FAQs about Intermittent Fasting

The practice of fasting just on certain days is fraught with misunderstandings. People who are unfamiliar with the process of fasting naturally have the tendency to express skepticism regardingthe health benefits associated with voluntarily abstaining from eating. The following is a collectionof responses to some of the most often asked questions and the most enduring myths regardingintermittent fasting.

10.1 Will My Body Go Into Starvation Mode?

One of the most common fears among those who are just starting out with intermittent fasting is the possibility of going into starvation mode. It should be made clear that starving mode, also known as adaptive thermogenesis, is a real phenomenon; yet, the process by which it operates is frequently misinterpreted.

If your body has an urgent need for energy, it will use the food you eat to meet that requirement,but any excess will be stored as fat for later use. You will put on weight if the amount of calories that enter the fat tissue is higher than the number of calories that exit the fat tissue. In the event that the contrary occurs, you will experience fat loss. The concept of "calories in, calories out" is founded on this observation (although the science is becoming more and more clear that not all calories are created equal). When you are attempting to lose weight, one of the most common things you will do is cut back on calories. This causes an imbalance between the number of calories you consume and the number of calories you burn, which will likely result in weight loss for you. You regard this as a positive, but your body views it as a negative influence on its health.

When you start to burn off extra calories and lose fat in the process, your body sees this as a threat since it is the beginning of an imminent hunger, and it reacts accordingly. The survival of your body is its primary priority. As a consequence of this, in an attempt to save itself, your bodybegins to conserve calories and does not burn them off as effectively, which causes your calorieneeds to decrease over time and especially after a considerable amount of weight reduction. This process is referred to as adaptive thermogenesis.

10.2 Norepinephrine: what exactly is it?

Norepinephrine, commonly known as noradrenaline, is a chemical found in the human body that is a member of the catecholamine family. The sympathetic nervous system is responsible for its release into the bloodstream in reaction to anything that the brain interprets as being in a stressfulsituation. The discharge of norepinephrine accelerates reaction times, raises blood flow, and causes an increase in the release of glucose into the bloodstream. It also causes an increase in the heart rate. The neurotransmitter is an essential component of the body's fight-or-flight response when faced with a potentially dangerous situation.

Many individuals are of the opinion that eating several smaller meals throughout the day is the best way to prevent the body from going into famine mode. It is for this reason that you are likelyto have heard the piece of advice that it is preferable to consume five or six smaller meals throughout the day rather than two or three larger meals. However, despite the fact that adaptivethermogenesis is a true process, it does not work exactly in that way. It is only when you go without food for an extended amount of time, such as days or weeks, rather than for a shorter period of time, such as hours, that your body will reach a state of real famine.

In the event that the body slipped into hunger mode within a short period of time, it would be extremely detrimental to the continuation of the human species. It would have been more difficultto hunt and gather food during the Paleolithic era if one's metabolism slowed down, which wouldhave led to a reduction in one's overall energy levels. If those who hunted and gathered didn't have access to food, their metabolism would slow down even further, their energy levels would continue to decrease, and they would eventually be unable to stay alive.

According to a number of studies, the practice of intermittent fasting does not hinder your body's ability to get rid of excess calories and fat; in fact, it has the opposite effect on your metabolic rate. The amount of calories you burn at rest, also known as your basal metabolic rate (or BMR),is said to increase by a significant amount when you incorporate short-term fasting, according to research that was published in The American Journal of Clinical Nutrition and The American Journal of Physiology. The reason for this is due to the fact that when you enter a fasting state, the levels of the hormone and neurotransmitter norepinephrine in your blood decrease. Norepinephrine is a stress hormone. This revs up your metabolism and sends a signal to your body to start shedding the excess body fat it has stored.

10.3 When you fast, do you not experience a loss of muscle?

It is a widely held misconception that if you go too long without eating, your body will immediatelystart using your muscles as a source of energy. However, as a result of human evolution, this is not how things actually function.

In order for the body to accomplish its primary objective, which is to survive, it has to get energy.It derives most of its supply from glucose, which is primarily derived from carbs. In the event that glucose is not there, the body will switch to using fat, which is essentially just energy that has been stored. Keep in mind that if you consume more calories than your body needs, it will convertthose extra calories into triglycerides and store those triglycerides in the fat cells of your body. When glucose levels and fat levels in the body drop to dangerously low levels, the body will naturally start breaking down muscle tissue for use as a source of energy.

This condition can only arise when the percentage of fat in the body falls below 4%, which is a very low level. To put this into perspective, the average body fat percentage for male athletes is between 6 and 13 percent, while the average body fat percentage for female athletes is between14 and 20 percent. Your muscles will remain intact until your body fat level drops to the point

Where they have no other alternative but to be used as a source of energy. The vast majority of people never get to this point.

It is true that if you reduce your calorie intake without engaging in any kind of resistance training,there is a probability that you will experience some loss of muscle mass; nevertheless, fasting does not make the amount of muscle mass that you lose any more severe.

People who incorporate fasting into their attempt to lose weight have less of a drop in lean muscle mass than those who do not intermittently fast. This finding is supported by studies.

10.4 Will My Glucose Levels Get Dangerously Low?

Concerns regarding one's blood sugar level are among the most prevalent when it comes to the practice of intermittent fasting. If you've ever gone too long without eating, you've definitely felt the symptoms of low blood sugar, which include hunger, irritability, weakness, sweaty palms, and anxiety. At some point in your life, you've probably encountered these symptoms. It is not the fact that you have gone too long without eating that causes your blood sugar to drop too low; rather, it is the food that you had during the most recent meal that is responsible for causing your blood sugar to drop to an unsafe level.

When you have a meal that is high in carbohydrates, your bloodstream will experience a surge of glucose as a result of the meal. In response to the surge in glucose, your body secretes insulin, which transports the glucose into the cells so that it may be used as a source of energy. The more your glucose jumps, the greater the amount of insulin that is released; the greater the amount of insulin that is released, the more your blood sugar will drop over the course of time. When you combine fasting with a healthy diet that is moderate in carbohydrates to low in carbohydrates, your body becomes extremely efficient at managing blood glucose levels on its own. As a result,even when you go for an extended period of time without eating, you do not experience the dramatic spikes and dips in your blood sugar that are associated with not eating.

If you have trouble controlling your blood sugar or if you have diabetes, the glucose and insulin response doesn't function as effectively. Because of this, you should be sure to speak with your healthcare practitioner before beginning any form of fast to establish if it is appropriate for you.

10.5 Does Fasting Make You More Prone to Bingeing?

It is a common misconception that if you go too long without eating, whenever you do eat, you will overeat unhealthy foods and, as a result, put on weight. It's not as cut and dry as you may think; there are many aspects to take into account.

Studies on fasting every other day suggest that people who fast have a tendency to take in morecalories on the day following a twenty-four-hour fast, although the increase is less than 500 calories. This is due to the fact that people who fast are more hungry on the day after a fast. If you subtract the number of calories you would have consumed during the fast from the number of calories you would have consumed the next day with only a slight increase, you would still bein a calorie deficit.

The sudden drop in blood sugar that follows a meal that is high in carbohydrates, as well as an addiction to carbohydrates, are two common factors that contribute to the feeling of wanting to binge eat. After a certain amount of time spent practicing intermittent fasting, you will find that your feelings of hunger become more manageable, and you will have less of a desire to consume an excessive amount of food.

It is likely that persons who have struggled in the past with bulimia or binge-eating disorder wouldexperience binges or bulimic behavior as a result of fasting. If you have a history of disordered eating, you should make an appointment with your primary care physician before beginning an intermittent fasting regimen.

10.6 When is the Best Time to Work Out While I'm Fasting?

In the realm of fitness, there is an age-old argument concerning whether or not it is more beneficialto exercise when in a fasted condition (with an empty stomach) or while in a fed state (with a fullstomach) (a fed state). The answer is that it is contingent upon the level of exertion that you are performing. There are a number of advantages to working out when fasted; however, if you are an endurance athlete or you engage in high-intensity activity, it is possible that working out after you have eaten will be more beneficial for you.

When you workout, your body requires a greater amount of energy than it would normally require.The glucose that's already in your blood will be the first source of fuel that your body uses. As soon as that is depleted, it will begin to burn glycogen, which is a kind of glucose that is stored inthe liver. However, the increased energy demand that exercise places on the body will result in afaster depletion of glycogen because the liver stores enough glycogen to sustain your body's energy needs for twenty-four hours even in the absence of food. In general, your liver stores enough glycogen to sustain your body's energy needs for twenty-four hours even in the absenceof food. The amount of glycogen that is used up during exercise is proportional to both the lengthand the intensity of the activity that is being performed.

As soon as glycogen stores are depleted, the body shifts from utilizing carbs as a source of energyto utilizing fat instead. Both abstaining from food and engaging in vigorous physical activity stimulate the sympathetic nervous system, which in turn controls the rate at which your body metabolizes fat. Combining the two significantly boosts the efficiency of the physiological systemsthat are responsible for converting fat into usable energy. In contrast to glycogen, which can onlybe stored in limited quantities, your body is able to store a limitless quantity of fat; therefore, youwill never run out. Your muscles will gradually become accustomed to utilizing whatsoever sourceof energy you provide for them.

The quick onset of exhaustion and loss of energy that follows the depletion of all glycogen storesis referred to as "hitting the wall" or "bonking." This phenomenon is also known as "bonking." This

occurs frequently among athletes who compete in long-distance events, such as marathon runners and triathletes.

In a study that was published in the International Journal of Sport Nutrition and Exercise Metabolism, the researchers split 19 male participants evenly between two groups. When one group of men performed their aerobic activity (cardio) while they were in a fasted state, the othergroup of men performed their cardio while they were in a fed state. During each session of exercise, the participants had their heights and weights measured, completed a questionnaire about their eating habits, and submitted samples of their blood and urine.

After the conclusion of the research project, the scientists found that although both groups of menin the study lost weight, only the men who fasted had a reduction in the proportion of body fat that they carried. To put it another way, even though the guys in the fed group dropped weight, the proportion of their bodies that were composed of fat remained the same.

Both restricting your caloric intake and engaging in strenuous physical activity place a beneficialstrain on your body. This helps your muscles become more robust and fights off the effects of aging on the muscular tissue. When your body is subjected to this kind of stress, it causes the release of brain-derived neurotrophic factor (BDNF) and muscle regulatory factors (MRFs). BDNFand MRFs are proteins that send signals to the brain to cause it to generate new neurons, and MRFs cause the muscles to generate new muscle cells.

The release of BDNF and MRFs, as well as the subsequent generation of new neurons and muscle cells, can help maintain your brain, neurons, and muscle fibers biologically young, boostbrain function, avoid depression, boost testosterone levels, and increase growth hormone levelsin the body.

10.6.1 Hormonal Advantages of Working Out While Fasting

Exercising on an empty stomach has been demonstrated to maximize health by improving levels of two specific hormones: insulin and growth hormone. This is in addition to increasing the amountof fat that is burned throughout the workout.

According to several studies, engaging in physical activity while fasting may have a beneficial impact on insulin sensitivity (the way the body responds to insulin). Consuming an excessive amount of food causes an increase in blood sugar, which, in turn, causes your body to be subjected to a continuous onslaught of insulin. This can, over time, lead to an excess of insulin inthe body, which in turn reduces the sensitivity of your cells to the hormone.

By engaging in physical activity while in a state of fasting, you are not only preventing your bodyfrom releasing insulin into the blood, but you are also allowing it to burn up any surplus insulin that it might have stored up. When your body has a healthy response to insulin, it makes it simplerto lose fat and boosts blood supply to muscles, making it easier to build muscle. This also makesit easier to lose fat overall. Exercise performed while fasting stimulates the synthesis of growth

hormone, which not only assists in the reduction of body fat and the development of new muscletissue but also enhances the health of the bones.

If you have diabetes, especially type 1 diabetes, it is imperative that you consult your healthcare practitioner before making any alterations to your normal exercise program. Fasting before exercising can cause a dip in insulin levels as well as a drop in glucose levels. This might be harmful for someone who is already taking diabetic medication or is unable to regulate insulin levels effectively.

After exercising, it is best to refrain from eating for at least sixty to ninety minutes, as this will maximize the benefits of the workout. It is a common misconception that in order to get the mostout of a workout, you need to consume a substantial amount of protein soon after finishing it. However, research has shown that delaying your next meal for an hour to an hour and a half afterexercising results in greater fat loss. This is because your metabolic rate is higher after exercise.

10.7 Tips for Exercise

Even though it may take some additional planning to get into the right groove when you're intermittent fasting, it's important that you keep a regular exercise routine even though it may takesome extra planning to get into the right groove. Regular exercise is an essential component of staying healthy. Although the most important thing is to pay attention to what your body requiresspecifically, there are some general guidelines that can help you get started in designing your strategy.

10.7.1 Perform Exercises of a Low Intensity While You Are Fasting

Because the glycogen stores in your body are drained when you are in a fasting state, it is highlyunlikely that you will have the stamina to engage in high-intensity exercise at this time. When youexercise when you are fasting, you should limit yourself to activities with a lower intensity, such as strolling, yoga, or elliptical training. If you are trying to maximize the likelihood that your body will use protein as fuel while you are fasting, you should limit your workouts to those that last onehour or less. Endurance activity, such as jogging for several hours, is an example of this.

10.7.2 Perform Strenuous Physical Activity in a Fed State

On the days that you want to engage in high-intensity exercise, such as HIIT (or High-Intensity Interval Training: a type of workout in which you alternate short bursts of high-intensity exercise with longer periods of lower intensity exercise), or strength training, plan your workouts so that they take place within a few hours of a meal. This will help you maintain your energy levels throughout your workout. You provide your body the glucose and glycogen it needs to power youthrough your exercises if you work out after you've eaten, so that you're exercising in a nourished condition. Both a drop in blood sugar level and the loss of muscle mass can be avoided by doingthis.

The talk test is an effective method for determining how strenuous an exercise program is. Duringa workout of moderate intensity, you should find it rather easy to carry on a conversation with someone else. You should only be able to say a few words at a time when you are in a comfortablestate when performing high-intensity activity. You know you're pushing yourself too hard when you can't even have a conversation with someone while you're working out without becoming out of breath.

10.7.3 Timing Is Everything

Every strength-training session should take place in the window of time between two meals if your goal is to pack on some substantial muscle. After a session of strength training, your muscles need amino acids in order to grow and repair themselves; therefore, if gaining muscle is one of your goals, you should consume a meal high in protein one hour before your strength training session, as well as another meal high in protein sixty to ninety minutes after your workout is complete. At each meal, you should strive to consume between 20 and 30 grams of high-quality protein, as recommended by the Academy of Nutrition and Dietetics.

Bear in mind that the majority of people easily consume considerably in excess of the daily recommended amount of protein, so there is no need to go completely overboard with your consumption of protein. In order to provide you with some context, a chicken breast that is 6 ounces provides 52 grams of protein.

Branched-chain amino acids are a type of amino acid that can be used as a supplement if you are concerned about losing muscle when you are working out (BCAAs). Leucine, isoleucine, and valine are the three branched-chain amino acids that make up 35 percent of your muscle protein. Before you begin your workout, it is helpful to take a supplement containing between 5 and 10 grams of BCAAs. This will assist avoid muscle breakdown.

10.8 Can I eat whatever I want?

A ketogenic diet or a Paleo-style nutritional regimen is followed by many people who participate in intermittent fasting, however adhering to either of these diets is not required for success. It is up to you to choose which method of eating is most beneficial to your health, and getting to that point may need some trial and error. This cookbook does not contain any recipes that contain gluten, refined sugar, or soy products of any kind. When it comes to nutrition, the rule of thumb isthat the food should be as similar as possible to its natural state.

10.8.1 The Significance of Nutrients at the Micro level

The majority of the world's most popular diets place a strong emphasis on macronutrients (carbohydrates, protein, and fat). There are diets that are high in fat and low in carbohydrates, aswell as diets that are low in fat and high in carbohydrates. IIFYM stands for "if it fits your macros,"and it is based on the idea that you are free to eat whatever you want as long as you keep the proportion of carbohydrates, proteins, and fats that is optimal for your body. Another option is the"if it fits your micros" method. Even if some of these diets do place an emphasis on the quality of the food they consume, the vast majority of them are missing an important component of the health puzzle: micronutrients.

The term "macronutrient" comes from the fact that the human body requires huge amounts of certain particular nutrients. On the other hand, micronutrients get their name from the fact that the body requires just trace amounts of them. In contrast to micronutrients, macronutrients supply the body with both nutrients and calories.

Macronutrients include dietary fats, proteins, and carbohydrates, whereas micronutrients include vitamins and minerals. However, despite the fact that the body only requires micronutrients in trace levels, this does not indicate that they are of any less significance. In point of fact, the significance of consuming sufficient quantities of micronutrients cannot be emphasized enough.

Micronutrients are comprised entirely of dietary components such as vitamins and minerals. There are thirteen vitamins and sixteen minerals that you need to consume in sufficient quantities on a daily basis in order to maintain your health. Each of these vitamins and minerals is responsible for carrying out essential bodily processes that are necessary to keep things working well in the body. For example, collagen, which is an essential component of your bones, joints, and skin, can work more effectively when vitamin C is present.

Vitamin D is essential to the proper functioning of your immune system and also helps strengthen your bones. Together, sodium and potassium are responsible for regulating the fluid and electrolyte balance in the body. Your ability to correctly digest carbs, proteins, and lipids is madepossible by the B vitamins. Additionally, vitamin B6 helps in the production of new blood cells andneurotransmitters in the body.

Vitamin A is essential for proper color vision as well as vision in low-light conditions. If you don't have enough vitamin K, your blood won't clot the right way. Calcium is responsible for the contraction of your muscles and enables nerves to communicate with one another. Obviously, this merely scratches the surface of the issue. There are an infinite number of additional functionsthat these and several other vitamins and minerals perform. Magnesium is responsible for more than three hundred different chemical processes in the body by itself.

If you do not get enough of certain vitamins and minerals in your diet, you will eventually developa shortfall in those nutrients. Even a slight shortfall in just one micronutrient can result in significant negative effects on one's health, despite the fact that it may not appear to be a significant issue. Low levels of vitamin D, for instance, have been linked to a number of mental health conditions, including depression (particularly seasonal affective disorder, which manifests itself during the winter months), as well as irritable bowel syndrome.

Magnesium shortage can lead to abnormal heartbeat, twitching and cramping of the muscles, elevated blood pressure, weariness, melancholy, and apathy (lack of emotion). Anemia, tingling in the hands and feet, exhaustion, weakness, irritability, and depression are some of thesymptoms that can result from not getting enough vitamin B12. Dementia, psychosis, and

Significant depression are some of the mental diseases that might manifest themselves if a B12 deficiency progresses to a severe enough level.

These impacts are concerning and have the potential to be fairly catastrophic, and research demonstrates that the majority of people are lacking in at least one micronutrient. According to the findings of the United States Department of Agriculture (USDA), the majority of adult Americans do not get sufficient amounts of calcium, potassium, magnesium, vitamin A, vitamin C, vitamin D, and vitamin E through their daily diets.

Seventy different dietary intakes from a group of men and women were analyzed in a study that was published in the Journal of the International Society of Sports Nutrition. The study found thaton average, males' diets were lacking in forty percent of the vitamins and just over fifty-four percent of the minerals. Although the diets of the ladies were marginally better than those of the males, they were still lacking in 29 percent of the vitamins and just over 44 percent of the minerals.

Although there aren't any hard-and-fast guidelines for what you should consume during meals when you're doing intermittent fasting, eating a balanced diet that includes a wide variety of fruits and vegetables and limits nutrient-deficient foods like processed and packaged foods is the bestway to get adequate amounts of each micronutrient and prevent micronutrient deficiencies. Although there aren't any rules regarding what you should consume during meals when you're doing intermittent fasting.

10.8.11 Consuming Food Consciously

It is not appropriate to have a meal while working at your desk or driving between errands; rather,a meal ought to be something that is savored and enjoyed in its entirety. Eating slowly and attentively allows you to savor each mouthful and tune into the cues your body sends you to let you know when you've had enough to eat. This is an important component of maintaining good health. When you engage in intermittent fasting, you will have less opportunities to have meals throughout the day. This provides you with an even greater incentive to take things more slowly and savor the experience.

10.8.3 Mindful eating

Consider each of your meals to be an essential component of your day, rather than an afterthought to be completed as quickly as possible. When it's time to eat, put an end to everythingelse and make yourself comfortable for a meal the way it should be eaten. Take a few slow, deepbreaths and bring yourself into a state of relaxation to get your body ready for the digesting process.

According to research, people who eat when distracted, such as when sitting in front of the television, miss critical indications from the body that signal satiety. As a result, these individualsconsume more food than they would if they were eating without any distractions.

Eating with awareness is a terrific approach to learn how to pay attention to cues from your bodyand to practice maintaining a healthy balance. To get you started, here are some pointers to consider:

1. You are not responsible for cleaning your plate. You learn at a young age that it is proper etiquette to finish everything on your plate. It's possible that someone cautioned you against wasting food or reminded you that there are children in other areas of the world who would give anything for a warm dinner. Even though those words are intended to have a positive impact, there is a possibility that they will have the opposite effect in the long run.

You may have a tendency to consume every morsel of food on your plate, even if you're full halfway through the meal, if those attitudes were instilled in you as a child and carried into adulthood. This is not to mean that you should be wasteful with food; nevertheless, rather than overeating in an effort to clean your plate, serve yourself a smaller piece to begin with, or reservewhat you are unable to finish for the following meal. Pay attention to your body and the cues it sends to let you know when you've had enough to eat, and then act accordingly.

2. Opt for Smaller Plates. It's possible that it's just a trick of the mind, but using a smaller plate can actually help you restrict the amount of food you eat. When you have a plate in your hand, you naturally want to fill it. This indicates that when you have a large plate, you will normally serveyourself more food than you would if you had a smaller plate. If you had a smaller plate, you wouldserve yourself less food. Choose to serve your meal on a salad or appetizer dish rather than a dinner plate. If you are still hungry after the first helping, you may always go back for seconds, but you should give yourself some time to let your food settle first.

3. Put Your Utensils Aside Between Each Bite. The mentality of today's society is "go, go, go."People have a tendency to speed through their entire days, including the time they spend eating.Take a deep breath and savor the moment the next time you sit down to eat a meal. Put down your fork in between bites and chew your food thoroughly rather than speeding through the mealand trying to gulp down each bite as quickly as possible.

4. Make sure to pay attention. When was the last time you paid attention to the texture of the food you were eating? When was the last time you even thought about it? When you're in a hurryto get to the next moment, it's easy to rush through your meal and not pay attention to the little things like the crunch of almonds in your lips, the tanginess of your salad dressing, or the coolnessof a piece of avocado. It is important to make it a point to pay attention to the entire experience, not just the taste of the meal you are eating. Consuming food is supposed to be an enjoyable experience. Take everything in.

10.9 Isn't it unhealthy for women to go without food?

It is a widely held misconception that women should not fast because it is detrimental to their health. While this may be the case for some women, it is not a generalization that can be made for all women. This hypothesis came about because intermittent fasting has the potential to induce

a hormonal imbalance in some women if the fasting is not done properly. However, when the rightcare and precautions are taken, women are able to fast successfully. This led to the developmentof this theory.

Women are more susceptible to the effects of possible malnutrition than males are since their bodies were anatomically and biologically intended to carry infants. In the event that a woman's body detects that she is about to go hungry, it will react by elevating her levels of the hormones leptin and ghrelin, which are responsible for regulating appetite. Even if a woman is not pregnantat the moment, her body will respond with this hormone reaction in order to safeguard a fetus thatis in the process of growing.

Even though it is feasible to ignore the hunger signals from ghrelin and leptin, doing so becomesprogressively difficult when the body rebels and begins to create more of these hormones. This is especially true when the body is in a state of starvation. If a woman gives in to her hunger in amanner that is detrimental to her health, such as by overeating or ingesting foods that are detrimental to her health, this might set off a chain reaction of additional hormonal disorders withinsulin.

This procedure has the potential to disable the reproductive system as well. If your body believesthat it does not have enough food to survive, it may stop the capacity to conceive in order to safeguard a possible pregnancy. Because of this, women who are pregnant or who are attemptingto conceive should not fast, and neither should women who are not pregnant.

The hypothalamic-pituitary-gonadal axis, often known as the HPG axis, is responsible forcontrolling the endocrine glands that are involved in the process of ovulation. The hypothalamus is responsible for the initial step in the ovulation process, which is the release of gonadotropin releasing hormone, also known as GnRH. Following the discharge of GnRH, the pituitary gland responds by discharging both follicle-stimulating hormone (also known as FSH) and luteinizing hormone (LH).

The release of follicle stimulating hormone (FSH) and luteinizing hormone (LH) in women is whattriggers the ovaries to produce estrogen and progesterone. It is the rise in estrogen and progesterone levels that ultimately leads to the maturation and subsequent release of an egg (ovulation). This hormonal cascade is quite precise and well-defined, and it occurs in a predictablepattern in women who are otherwise healthy. Fasting, on the other hand, can throw off GnRH levels because of its great sensitivity to the environment and other external factors.

Even though it operates in a somewhat different way, men also have an HPG axis in their bodies.Both FSH and LH are responsible for stimulating the creation of testosterone and sperm, but theydo so via acting on the testes rather than the ovaries, which are absent in males. However, because men's bodies were not intended to carry offspring, the HPG axis in males is not as sensitive to the effects of fasting as it is in women. As a result, the protection alert that the body has is not triggered as quickly.

10.9.1 Crescendo Fasting

If you are a woman, this does not imply that intermittent fasting is not appropriate for you; rather,it indicates that you should ease into it more gently and proceed with caution. You may choose to begin with crescendo fasting if you are a lady who is attempting fasting for the first time to determine if it is something that you should continue doing.

Instead of fasting for twelve to sixteen hours each and every day, crescendo fasting requires youto limit your fasting to only a few days per week for a few days per week. These days of abstinenceshould not be consecutive (Tuesday, Thursday, and Saturday, for example). On days when you are fasting, you should limit your physical activity to light activities such as walking or yoga. On non-fasting days, when you are eating regularly and not restricting your calories, strength trainingand other strenuous forms of activity should be avoided.

It is also essential to consume a large amount of water every day. The standard advice is the ounces' equal of half of your body weight; for example, if you weigh 280 pounds, you should consume a minimum of 70 ounces of water on a daily basis. You should use this equation as a starting point because the amount of water you require is contingent on a wide range of parameters, including your age, weight, activity level, and the quantity of coffee you consume; nonetheless, you should still utilize this equation.

If you feel good after progressively fasting for a couple of weeks, you can throw in another day offasting and see how your body reacts to the increased amount of time spent without eating. If youare still in good health, you can extend your fast for additional days until you reach the number ofdays you have set for yourself. The body should not be shocked all at once, as this defeats the purpose of crescendo fasting, which is to wean off of food gradually.

Conclusion

I n conclusion, it is clear that intermittent fasting can be a highly effective tool for women looking to improve their overall health and reach their weight loss goals. By restricting their eating window and allowing their bodies to enter a fasted state, women can experience a wide range of benefits, including weight loss, improved insulin sensitivity, and increased mental clarity. Additionally, intermittent fasting is often easier to adhere to than traditional dietary plans and can be used to break through weight loss plateaus. Ultimately, the choice of whether to incorporate intermittent fasting into one's lifestyle is a personal one that should be based on an individual's goals and preferences.

Throughout the course of this book, we have thoroughly examined the various types of intermittent fasting that are available and how they can be tailored to fit the unique needs and lifestyle of each individual woman. We have also delved into the potential benefits and drawbacks of intermittent fasting and provided valuable tips and strategies for successful implementation. With the information within this book, you should now have the tools necessary to make an informed decision about whether intermittent fasting is right for you.

If after reading this book, you decide that intermittent fasting is right for you, then you can start implementing it right away and enjoying the potential benefits it can bring. If you find that intermittent fasting is not for you, then you should feel comfortable continuing to pursue a healthylifestyle without it. Whatever your decision, make sure to listen to your body and take care of yourself.

One of the most crucial messages that has been emphasized throughout this book is the importance of finding a fasting protocol that works best for you. It is important to remember that intermittent fasting is not a one-size-fits-all approach, and it is necessary to experiment and see what works best for your body, lifestyle, and individual preferences. Additionally, it is important to listen to your body while implementing the fasting protocol and make any necessary adjustmentsalong the way. This could include adjusting the fasting window or taking breaks from fasting if needed.

Furthermore, it is essential to make sure that your overall diet is nutritionally balanced and contains a wide variety of healthy whole foods to ensure that you are getting all of the micronutrients and vitamins your body needs for optimal health. Moreover, it is important to incorporate physical activity into your routine to ensure that you are getting the exercise your bodyneeds to remain healthy.

With the right combination of these elements, intermittent fasting can bea highly effective tool for women looking to improve their overall health and reach their weight loss goals.

In fulfilling our promise to provide a solution for the reader, we have offered practical and actionable advice for incorporating intermittent fasting into your daily routine. We have also stressed the importance of maintaining a healthy and balanced diet, staying properly hydrated,

and getting enough sleep. These factors are all essential to achieving the maximum benefits of intermittent fasting and maintaining overall health and wellness.

With the information within this book, you should now have the tools necessary to make an informed decision about whether intermittent fasting is right for you. Ultimately, it is up to you to decide whether intermittent fasting is a lifestyle you wish to pursue.

One takeaway that we hope the reader will take away from this book is the understanding that intermittent fasting can be a powerful tool for improving health and achieving weight loss goals, but it is important to approach it with caution and seek guidance from a healthcare professional before starting any new diet or exercise program. It is also crucial to find a fasting protocol that works for you and to listen to your body's needs. With dedication and commitment, intermittent fasting can be a valuable addition to any woman's health and wellness journey.

The information in this book has been designed to provide you with the knowledge and resourcesnecessary to make an informed decision about intermittent fasting and whether it is right for you. With this information, you can start incorporating intermittent fasting into your routine and enjoy the potential benefits it can bring.

Finally, it is important to keep in mind that intermittent fasting is just one tool for improving overallhealth and reaching weight loss goals. Health and wellness should be a priority in all aspects of life, and it is important to recognize that a balanced diet and regular physical activity are also essential components of maintaining a healthy lifestyle. Additionally, it is important to prioritize self-care, get enough sleep, and find ways to reduce stress. By combining intermittent fasting with a well-balanced diet, regular physical activity, self-care habits, and stress-relief techniques, you can maximize the potential benefits of intermittent fasting and achieve your goals.

In conclusion, it is clear that intermittent fasting can be a highly effective tool for women looking to improve their overall health and reach their weight loss goals. By restricting their eating windowand allowing their bodies to enter a fasted state, women can experience a wide range of benefits, including weight loss, improved insulin sensitivity, and increased mental clarity. Additionally, intermittent fasting is often easier to adhere to than traditional dietary plans and can be used to break through weight loss plateaus.

Thank You!

Hope you've enjoyed your reading experience.

So, I'd like to thank you for supporting me and reading until the very end.

Before you go, would you mind leaving, a review?

It will mean a lot to me and support me in creating high-quality books, for you in the future.

Thanks once again and here's where you can leave a review:

Warmly yours,

Melissa May

Your Free Gift

Before you go any further, why not pick up a free gift from me to you?

WEIGHT LOSS QUIZ

If you're a woman interested in trying intermittent fasting to achieve your weight loss goals, it's essential to find the right number of calories for you to eat in order to see success. The good news is that you can easily determine the exact number of calories you need to eat based on your metabolism, activity level, and time frame using our quiz at the link provided. Simply follow the prompts and you'll have all the details you need to get started on your weight loss journey with intermittent fasting.

Scan here to learn how much you need to eat in order to achieve your goals.

Melissa May

Feel free to continue your journey with us, where you will find new resources, tools, blogs, and advanced notice of new books at...

http://www.booksandsummaries.com/

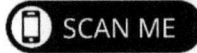

SCAN ME

www.ingramcontent.com/pod-product-compliance
Lightning Source LLC
Chambersburg PA
CBHW060459030426
42337CB00015B/1645